THE SKINNY ON EATING LIKE YOU GIVE A DAMN

HOW TO EMBRACE A PLANT-BASED DIET, COMBAT INJUSTICE, AND BE A REBEL FOR COMPASSION ONE BITE AT A TIME

D0877751

STEPHANIE HARTER

Award Winning Author

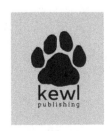

kewl
publishing

The Skinny On Eating Like You Give a Damn:
How to embrace a plant-based diet, Combat Injustice,
and Be a Rebel for Compassion One Bite at a Time

www.eatinglikeyougiveadamn.com

Copyright © 2019 by Stephanie Marie Linton Harter

All rights reserved. No portion of this book may be reproduced me-chanically, electronically, or by any other means, including photocopying, without permission of the publisher or author except in the case of brief quotations embodied in critical articles and reviews. It is illegal to copy this book, post it to a website, or distribute it by any other means without permission from the publisher or author.

Limits of Liability and Disclaimer of Warranty

The author and publisher shall not be liable for your misuse of this mate-rial. This book is strictly for informational and educational purposes. The information in this book is true and complete to the best of our knowl-edge. In no way is this book intended to replace, countermand, or conflict with the advice given to you by your own physician. The ultimate decision concerning care should be made between you and your doctor. The author and publisher disclaim all liability in connection with the use of this book.

The purpose of this book is to educate and entertain. The author and/or publisher do not guarantee that anyone following these techniques, sug-gestions, tips, ideas, or strategies will become successful. The author and/ or publisher shall have neither liability nor responsibility to anyone with respect to any loss or damage caused, or alleged to be caused, directly or indirectly by the information contained in this book.

Cover art design by Scott Lancaster and Dragan Bilic.
Photographs by Elizabeth Harden.

On the cover, Stephanie is featuring an Impossible Burger with Follow Your Heart dairy-free cheese alternative provided by Farmacy Vegan Kitchen & Bakery in Tampa, FL.

Testimonial submissions from the Eating Like You Give A Damn Facebook Community are published with permission by each contributor.

ISBN: 978-1-64184-060-6

Publisher
Kewl Publishing
Largo, FL
USA

Thank you for purchasing this book

A portion of the proceeds from your purchase of this book goes toward helping the efforts of Florida Rescue Farm who provide rehabilitation, relocation assistance, and a forever home to unwanted farm animals in southwestern Florida. Your contribution goes to feed, supplements, shelter and vet care, making a difference in the lives of the resident animals while supporting the farms educational efforts to enhance the lives of future generations.

Visit www.floridarescuefarm.org to learn more.

****

FREE BONUS DOWNLOAD

"The secret to getting ahead is getting started." Mark Twain

Go to www.eatinglikeyougiveadamn.com/guide

to download your **FREE COPY** of the

Eating Like You Give a Damn

Endless Plant-Based Food Guide

It is the companion to this book, and the only guide you'll ever need to decide what to eat every day - and the options are truly endless. It contains hyperlinks to the latest omnivore-approved meat, dairy, and egg replacements that you can find in your local grocery store, healthy whole food recommendations, and a customizable menu chock full of 100% plant-based foods using a variety of flavors so your vegan meals are never bland or boring.

****

Dedication

To the rebels of the world sharing the vision of a more compassionate and just world for all, whether in your business, nonprofit work, or at the dinner table. I truly believe you hold the key to peace for all who inhabit the earth by breaking the widespread dependency on animal products through your positive work and leadership. You are forever my inspiration.

And, to my husband, Dave - the strongest, sexiest, and most supportive man with the kindest heart I have ever known. You are my rock, and I love you more.

Table of Contents

Introduction

"Our lives begin to end the day we become silent about things that matter." Dr. Martin Luther King, Jr.

Rebels are visionaries. They see the world for what it is, and are forever leading the way to how it could be. This is not out of some morally superior need to be cooler than everyone else, as one might think. Indeed, quite the contrary.

Rebels have traditionally been viewed as misunderstood hell-raising misfits, yet throughout history we have experienced significant revelations in the way we view one another, and the revolutions that have come of it. Rebels are everywhere rejecting the status quo, combating injustice, and leading the charge to social changes that make a difference.

As you will learn in this book, the problem we face today is that we are in the thick of a global crisis that no one wants to have a constructive conversation around, whether on the news, in our workplaces, or at the dinner table. Yet, it affects every single one of us on the planet. And it starts with what's at the end of our forks.

On one hand, we have officials who operate the food system like health isn't their problem, yet we rely on the very corporations that are producing the very foods that create the problems to educate the public about our "health." And on the other hand, we have a healthcare system that enables pharmaceuticals and invasive surgeries like *what we eat* isn't the problem, or more specifically, our *solution.*

More people are recognizing today that these systems are causing extreme problems with millions of people suffering from preventable disease, billions of animals tortured and slaughtered, and the Earth's resources being destroyed so rapidly that we are driving full speed into extinction...for a profit. The very foods that are causing all this havoc are viewed by the masses as normal, natural and necessary, and they're even subsidized by governments.

That's right fellow taxpayers. We're being bamboozled, and it's costing us big time. And in case you've been away on another planet and this is your first time hearing it, I'm talking about meat, dairy, eggs and other animal by-products.

Profits generated from animal agribusiness are regarded as more important than people's health, more important than the environment, and more important than the people's right to transparency about how our food is being produced.

So, is this a hopeless situation? Absolutely not, because we - the consumers - have the power to shift economics into a more favorable outcome for all by simply displacing the money we spend on meat, dairy, and eggs onto the hundreds of other plant-based options available to us. And, the United Nations urges us to do so before our time runs out.

We're currently on the verge of a global uprising of rebels vying for a more compassionate and just food system. And the rivals? Some might say "meat-eaters" but I don't agree - I say follow the money and the rivals will appear. Because, *I* was once a meat-eater. I ate burgers smothered in cheese and washed it down with a big glass of milk once upon a time, and I believed it to be normal and without consequences. I've since had a wakeup call, and it felt something like choosing the red pill and seeing The Matrix for what it really was. I went deep down the rabbit hole for truth and validity, and it changed how I show up in the world today: as a *rebel for compassion*.

I was happy to discover that not only was I in good company with other rebels all over the world leading the movement to ending the suffering caused by animal agribusiness, but also that eliminating animal products from the human diet is supported by thousands of medical research studies; making any animal who ends up on a dinner plate an unnecessary commodity.

A rebel for compassion is different from what the majority assumes all "vegans" to be. A rebel for compassion is a benevolent disruptor who lives by their values and speaks up where they see injustice towards people and animals. They have a respected presence, and not because they're boisterous, but because of their extraordinary ability to understand where the problem persists, and bravely go against the grain in order to build the bridge over to the solution.

A rebel for compassion leads with warmth and gratitude, cultivating trust because people understand that their ego has nothing to do with the mission. Through authenticity, empathy, knowledge, passion, and charisma, a rebel for compassion possesses the influence to make the world take notice. They are the catalyst for social change, and they lift up others to support a collective success in the creation of a just system for people and animals.

My purpose for this book is to help you catch the vision of your true freedom, and to follow my actionable guide for adopting healthy change and living joyfully as an effective advocate for animals, the planet, and each other. And, so that you may find others to relate to other than me, some of the members of the Eating Like You Give a Damn community on Facebook have provided their insights within the chapters as well.

Eating Like You Give a Damn is the way that you can take action on the philosophy that good food can be enjoyed without dire consequences. Thank you for saying Yes to the exploration of one of the most misunderstood topics of our time, and discovering how to thrive as a rebel for compassion.

Veg On, Rebel.

Stephanie

1

Betty Crocker to Veggie Rocker

"First they ignore you, then they laugh at you, then they fight you, then you win." Mahatma Gandhi

My friends and family didn't notice me rocking my latest cruelty-free makeup, notice me reducing my overall plastic use, or comment on the process of me transitioning to eco-friendly clothing and household products. It's also not likely that they saw the fair trade symbol on the coffee I switched to, the biodegradable straws I've adopted, or that I have donated my time and money to a local animal sanctuary.

But what they did notice right away is that I had stopped eating what I was normally used to eating. Meat. Dairy. Eggs. Three kinds of food which everyone around me had an unshakable attachment to. And that, at times, became the topic of conversation in which I felt like I was being held in contempt.

It was an interesting conundrum when it happened because, from my perspective, I remember fellow associates had applauded me in the past for exhibiting compassion towards others, my commitment to taking responsibility for my health through exercise and mindful eating, and they even awed at my displays of affection for animals.

And then, when they realized I had a change of heart about eating the animals that were once on my plate, it seemed to me at times like it was taken as a judgement on their behavior even though I never indicated any such thought.

I found myself under a blanket of fast-firing questions and snarky remarks while I was still in the process of trying to figure it all out for myself.

I had come to the conclusion after much deliberation that the case against eating animals and their by-products (i.e. eggs, milk) is strong on health, moral, and environmental grounds, yet my patience and resilience was being tested daily from the time my feet touched the floor up until they were tucked back into the covers and lights out.

During my journey in finding my way to eating what my conscience allowed, I had a moment of sheer clarity in realizing that eating animals wasn't for me for a variety of reasons. I didn't reach this decision easily, or overnight. It was through careful thought and consideration, and in spite of that fact, the world seemed to be on a mission to derail my efforts of living more in alignment with my values.

There were many times my mind would spin with ways that I could have handled certain comments and criticisms better, but in the moment when they launched that question or comment, I felt emotional, annoyed, or caught off guard completely. I realized many of my knee-jerk responses may as well have sealed my doom as the most ineffective advocate for health and the movement toward compassionate social change.

I didn't sign up to evangelize or be the next poster child for veganism. Heck, I avoided even labeling myself as *anything* that puts moral ideology into a neat little box for fear of being judged wrongly by people who criticize what they don't understand. Many people tried to pull me back after falling out of the status quo while I watched them pulling cooked and seasoned animal flesh and fat off of bone fragments butchered from a once living, breathing, feeling animal with their teeth, and neatly slicing their steak into bite sized pieces as they declared that humans were meant to eat meat. Just like I used to do and believe. Until one day, I felt a twinge of responsibility to set the record straight.

Before I embarked on the quest to finding out the real deal about meat, dairy and eggs, where they actually come from and why we eat them, I assumed I already knew the answers. However, this was not the case. What I uncovered affected more than just the animals that I wanted to save. It appears that the general population, whether having an affinity towards animals or not, would find it unusual or extreme to give those privileged foods up. Yet, they don't know the whole truth. And, those who once ate animals and have shifted to a vegan lifestyle suspect that if they did, they would care enough to change some of their eating habits too.

The truths that were uncovered once I was ready and willing to receive the full story behind the widespread practice of animal exploitation smacked me hard on my ass, leaving me feeling betrayed by anyone who told me it was normal, healthy and necessary to eat animals.

I felt like the consequences of eating animals, dairy and eggs was more shocking and detrimental to our population than focusing all our attention on GMOs and the harmful chemicals in our non-organic foods. Yet, all the welcome buzz in my local grocery store focused on local, organic, sustainable, grass-fed, free range, wild caught and humane meat, dairy and eggs - and *not* the truth of the many health and environmental repercussions involved with raising and eating them at all.

Based on certain evidence, some of which I include in this book, I feel that it is more life threatening and destructive for our shared planet to consume animal products than all the buzz online about cleansing, dieting, detoxing, and debating less impactful topics, like whether or not coconut oil is good for you.

Meanwhile, meat, dairy and eggs are proven contributors to deadly heart disease, stroke, diabetes, Alzheimer's, auto-immune diseases, hypertension and cancer, which many of us see our loved ones afflicted with and once assumed was simply genetic.

Even the World Health Organization has classified all mammalian muscle meat, including, beef, veal, pork, lamb, mutton, horse, and goat, as a Group 2 carcinogen. And pro-cessed meats, such as sausages, ham, lunch meat, canned meat, jerky, hot dogs, and yes...bacon, are classified as Group 1 car-cinogens, which is the same cancer-causing class as cigarettes.

Animal agriculture is the leading cause of species extinc-tion, deforestation, climate change, illness-inducing pollution, antibiotic resistance, and deplorable breeding, confinement and killing practices of the animals we label as food.

And it's literally killing people, one preventable disease after another.

Furthermore, over 70% of the ocean's fish species are either fully exploited or depleted while delicate ecosystems that have existed since prehistoric times have been destroyed by the fishing industry. Not to mention the millions of deaths of turtles, dolphins, whales, birds, rays, and other non-targeted by-catch victims. Meanwhile, the farmed fish industry dumps GMOs and antibiotics into their fish feed, which end up in our freshwater.

When I got to the bottom of it, I was left at that time wondering if there was any hope left for humanity since the world I was experiencing seemed to be *against* and not *for* a plant-based lifestyle.

WTF?

Making of a Rebel

Most of my family hail from North Carolina and Virginia, so I grew eating the typical Southern American fare you'd find in a Betty Crocker Cookbook, and together with the recipes found inside the Campbell's Soup can labels, which I had loved and took comfort in my whole life.

I was raised on fried eggs in bacon grease, tuna sandwiches, spaghetti with giant meatballs, meatloaf and mashed potatoes with canned green beans, fried chicken, Kraft macaroni and cheese, and collards boiled with a ham hock. Just about everything was seasoned with a big dollop of Country Crock spread. Salad was my favorite side, so long as it was drenched in ranch dressing and sharp cheddar cheese. In fact, I used to joke that vegetables were just ranch dressing delivery devices. And for lunch almost every day, I ate deli cut meats and cheese on white toast.

My favorite casseroles were creamy tuna casserole, and chicken divan smothered in cream of mushroom sauce and cheddar cheese.

We visited various fast food drive-thrus on the regular, and my family's favorite restaurants included the 5 for $5 deals and the all you can eat buffets. Burgers, pizza and seafood alfredo were all time favorites when we were eating out at restaurants. Sprinkle in the nutritionally-void processed foods like Slurpees, cheese puffs, and Hostess snack cakes, and I now believe you get the picture.

When I was fifteen, there was a particular night at the dinner table with my mom, dad, little sister and baby brother when I remember sawing my knife through the middle of my steak and watching blood pool onto my plate. I immediately lost my appetite, but really didn't understand why, since it appeared that no one else seemed to mind seeing blood trickle from their beef. In a tongue in cheek sort of way while encouraging me to finish my dinner, my dad referenced the meat on my plate as "still mooing."

I shot back that the meat was not from a once living cow that moo'd, but grown from the ground like vegetables. At least, it's what I told myself in order to stuff down my natural reaction to the sudden conscious realization that a gentle creature had to die so I could eat this. Yet there I was, voicing it aloud. He giggled, not maniacally - just as a kind gesture to my delusion.

I knew just how ridiculous it sounded the moment the words passed from my lips. And, my mom and dad were pretty supportive of whatever I needed to convince myself of in order for me to finish my meal.

I concluded in that moment that my reaction, well-meaning as it may have seemed, was strange and unbefitting to any normal girl because eating certain animals *was* normal. After all, everyone I knew led me to believe this, and they all demonstrated to me just how normal and necessary it is. In fact, the TV had advertisements that said so, my schools and teachers said so, my athletic mentors, the advertisements everywhere in my magazines, the celebrities endorsing it, billboards, grocery stores, restaurant menus, and all of my family and friends. There were even posters plastered on the walls at my school naming the health benefits of eating meat, dairy and eggs, such as protein, calcium, and iron. These foods were advertised as the foundation for muscular strength, strong bones, healthy blood and overall energy. These were all things I knew I wanted, so it never occurred to me that any of those advertisements could be misleading.

This was my observation from the world around me, so it had to be right. I was fully immersed in the idea that it was necessary to get nutrients from meat, dairy and eggs, and was never cognizant that there might be another choice, in fact a choice I could make on my own.

I had never known anyone to contest it, so I did what any rule abiding teenager would do. I obeyed my dad, and I finished the final pieces of my rare steak. I took that conscious realization and tucked it neatly back where it belonged deep in my subconscious mind, where I hopefully would never have to encounter it again.

The next day, I was back to normal. I ate animals and their by-products for breakfast, lunch, and dinner. I continued to do so every day afterward, never again conjuring such thoughts about my food until later in life.

That was my earliest memory of breaking free from the cognitive dissonance we all experience, where my intrinsic beliefs about not harming anyone, including animals, were conflicting with my habit of eating only some of them. Additionally, I was unconscious to how it was negatively impacting me on many levels, including my health and my spirit.

As I reflect, I can recall many similar examples of bearing witness to everyday violence against animals. Like when I refused to dissect frogs and fetal pigs in my 10th grade biology honors class, and bearing the ridicule from my peers, and getting a D as my final grade.

And, when I was eighteen, I adopted a potbelly pig and named him Elvis. He was smarter and more loving than any dog I had known. I freaked out after I watched Elvis eat my boyfriend's bacon, which I realized might have been a distant cousin to my pet pig. Then it hit me...I had been eating someone else's Elvis. Eating one pig while petting another felt ever so wrong in that moment, yet, that didn't stop me. So I returned to the safety of the status quo.

And later, when I was twenty-one, I snuck away from my family's big Independence Day party to secretly experience my first petrifying panic attack at the sight of everyone picking flesh straight off of an entire pigs dead body laying inside of a smoker. I remember my breathing became shallow and I gasped for air. I gripped the edges of the bathroom counter to steady myself, but it felt as though I had no strength to hold myself up. My body trembled, my vision got dark and narrow, and my heart felt like it would burst from my chest. I was terrified I would be found later either unconscious or dead on the bathroom floor. Thankfully, I recovered. After fixing my makeup, I gathered my emotions, and went into the kitchen to take a couple of shots of tequila. Then, I went back out to the pig pickin' before anyone noticed I was really a social reject posing as a normal person.

I must confess also that there were strong feelings of remorse that would bubble up in me after witnessing and participating in the violent things everyday normal people would do. For instance, behead a garden snake they were afraid of, kill mice on glue traps for infiltrating their homes, hook and behead a writhing fish and proudly bringing it home for dinner, and dumping live crabs into a vat of boiling water while watching them try to crawl out, and then afterwards, smashing the shells of their bodies with hammers to retrieve and eat their meat. I was even repulsed by my own irrational violence against spiders.

Additionally, while my husband, Dave, and I were living in southern Italy as he was serving in the Navy, we rescued a very skittish ten-week-old puppy off of the dangerous streets and called her Lady. We were no strangers to rescued animals, as we already had adopted two others in our family (Stewie the cat, and Cannoli the dog). However, we did not intend to keep her. When we first found this scared puppy without a mother in sight, she resembled a common companion dog that many Americans wouldn't hesitate to rescue and give shelter to. However, she behaved as a terrified wild animal who practically slept with one eye open until she learned to trust that she was safe. During those pivotal first few months since we met, Lady had taught us more about trust, patience, courage and overwhelming gratitude than we had ever learned from any other source. While we initially fostered Lady with the intention of rehabilitating her for adoption into another good home, we developed an unbreakable family bond. So, we proudly flew this Italian street dog back to America with us to remain in our family forever. To this day, Lady is an incredibly loving, playful and protective companion animal who reminds us that when any animal is given the opportunity to express their individuality in a safe environment, even after experiencing trauma, they can teach us so much about our own humanity if we are willing and open to the lessons.

To some who accepts things as they are and are not connected to their intrinsic empathy for creatures who also feel emotional and physical pain the way that people do, coming to grips with giving up the "right" to eat animal-derived foods might be a far stretch.

That's why today, in the post-digital age where information is widely accessible from the palm of our hands or by asking Alexa, we are so very fortunate to be able to appeal to people's health and wellbeing as well as the future of the planet - if we fail to appeal to their empathy for all creatures in nature rather than just some (like dogs and cats).

We have the opportunity to open up more avenues for conversation around delicious plant-based food, health and the nonsensical use of animals as food sources than compassionate vegans once did, which explains why the plant-based and vegan movement has seen massive growth in just a few short years. And, it has only really just begun.

"I had spent almost 20 years as a lacto-ovo vegetarian. I was very happy with my decision and felt like I was doing my bit for the animals. I always thought that being vegan was so extreme and in all that time had absolutely no desire to become a vegan. I certainly didn't want to give up all my comfort foods, especially cheese and chocolate! I'm from the UK, and after living in the USA for about 1 year, I had gained a ton of weight, I felt very miserable and my health wasn't great. At this time my mum suffered from a stroke in her early 50's, and this shocked me to my core. I had to figure this out, for myself and for my family. I started researching all I could about health and in the process I learned about the detrimental effects that dairy, especially, can have on your health, so we hesitantly stopped giving my then 2-year-old son milk. This was so scary to me and my husband. We had been brought up to believe that cow's milk was a health food and that kids should have it in their diet. It was at this point that we went plant-strong but we still weren't committed vegans at this point. It was only after watching the documentary on Netflix called 'Food, Inc.' in floods of tears late one night that the reality of the animal cruelty that our meat and dairy industry are based upon hit me, like a bag of bricks in the face. That was the final straw, we became vegan that day, we never looked back and we are a very happy and healthy family who value life and health, of humans and animals alike. P.S., there is vegan cheese and chocolate, whew!"

Sara Day - Clearwater, FL

The End Game

There's a simple way for people to be healthy and happy without taking the life of an animal for food. So why wouldn't I live that way? That is the question I asked myself as I continued to learn more positive reasons for choosing a meatless burger over an animal-derived burger.

The reason I wrote this book is to inform you about the facts that I myself was surprised to uncover about eating animals and their by-products, and how your life could be improved should you choose to divorce yourself from them. You're going to learn:

- how our society perpetuates the myth that eating animals is necessary

- why we have a choice as omnivores to eat what our conscience allows

- and how to cross over to a healthier and more compassionate diet and lifestyle, even if you could never imagine giving up your favorite foods today.

And for the facts and reasons I provide from my education and experience, you will understand my passion for the topic and my joy for making Eating Like You Give a Damn the new normal in our society. But, don't just take my word for it. I encourage you to do your due diligence to uncover the hidden truths about animal agribusiness after reading this book, and then decide for yourself if becoming a rebel for compassion makes sense for you. Because, I believe that eating animals is a matter of personal choice *only after* all of the evidence regarding disease, animal exploitation, and the state of our environment has been fully examined.

While some people we encounter may hold limiting beliefs about how eating like you give a damn can make an impact, rebels who want to make a difference know what's at stake if action isn't taken to educate more people about their buying habits. For instance, it is not widely known that when we buy eggs, millions of baby male chicks are killed upon hatching because they don't produce those eggs; when we purchase dairy products, millions of newborn calves are turned into veal (if they're male) or become a vessel to produce milk (if they're female) as each mother cow bellows for the baby that was stripped from her care; when we buy meat, many chronic diseases are spread to other people from the billions of pounds of hog, cow, and chicken feces from concentrated animal feeding operations which contaminate our groundwater and air; and not only are modern ocean and freshwater fishing practices causing irreparable ecological havoc, the world's oceans are one of the primary reservoirs where the neurotoxin, mercury, is deposited and becomes biomagnified and bioaccumulated in seafood (according to Biodiversity Research Institute's 2014 report on Mercury in the Global Environment). This only scratches the surface of the great many issues that most people might have a strong emotional reaction to.

That being said, the act of rebelling against anything without communicating a well-defined end game isn't productive for getting people to change their habits. It's obvious that bringing the aforementioned injustices to a halt is the goal of many, and as such, vegans will tell you they want to see a vegan world. But the world needs to know exactly what that looks like in order to get on board with the notion. Achieving a vegan world is what many activists want on behalf of those without a voice. And, when you see so much wrong and you want more people to 'get woke' to what you believe is right, I believe we have to go beyond focusing on the problem. We have a responsibility to enroll people into the dream of what could be.

I hold a vision that when we open a menu at any mainstream restaurant, we will see every food our heart desires in the exact same way we see it today. From burgers, steaks, and fried chicken, to sushi, eggs benedict, and bacon wrapped anything. And here's the kicker...none of it will be derived from animals. Innovative foods replace the need to raise livestock or fish from the waters, and it will all have the same taste and texture of traditional meat, dairy, and egg products without the dire health consequences.

Animal agribusiness will no longer be a viable operation in this new economy where the demand for vegan food is high. And according to the United Nations, The Environmental Protection Agency, and The Environmental Working Group, not only is this possible, it's *necessary*.

As each operation converts to plant food production or closes altogether, workers are given the opportunity for new jobs with fewer health risks and hazardous conditions. The crops we farm to fatten livestock today could transition to crops that feed the nearly one billion people in the world who are chronically undernourished, and our fast growing future human population.

Millions of lives will be saved from diet related illness like heart disease, cancer and diabetes because plant-based foods are the predominant option by default. Money saved on healthcare costs boosts the economy and decreases poverty as health promoting produce is subsidized and made more affordable to everyone while supporting crop farmers.

Uncontaminated drinking water is available to everyone, leaving no cause for health concerns from polluted waters. And water and other vital resources are used in a sustainable way.

And when ocean dredging and large net fish gathering stops, underwater wildlife and ecosystems will flourish and no longer threaten collapse.

Air pollution dissipates, lessening the impact of weather related disasters like droughts, intense storms, and floods, and rain forests and wildlife flourish while the rate of species extinction slows to a stop.

The animals that were once used for their meat, bones, skins and organs for a profit find care and freedom from harm in a sanctuary.

Students learn in history books about how our generation saved the world, and they take field trips to nearby sanctuaries to meet the animal ambassadors.

I think then, we will experience a world where peace of mind and spirit exists on a massive scale.

It will take diligence, and it will take time. But the ball is already rolling in favor of a plant-based society. It won't be an overnight sensation, but as demand for animal products decreases, so too does the unnecessary production and oppression of those individual animals.

If we can imagine this brave new world, together we can achieve it. The revolution is here. As rebels for compassion, together, we will light the path to the solution so others may find their way to forming new food traditions. Together, we will reform the unsustainable and unjust systems perpetuated by animal agribusiness to improve the quality of our health, our world, and our humanity.

Are you ready to take on the role of a rebel? Good. Let's do this.

2

Wait, I've Been Bamboozled!

"Whenever you find yourself on the side of the majority, it's time to pause and reflect." Mark Twain

The simple act of choosing what we eat is the one thing we actively partake in three or more times daily, and in effect, this holds much responsibility in that it has such a profound impact on our personal health, our humanity, and the sustainability of our entire planet. So, why aren't more people aware of this?

More people are inclined to invest thousands of dollars into health and wellness products, as well as in aid for rescuing dogs and cats, and driving an electric car than they are in adopting a plant-exclusive lifestyle. Even though the latter proves to be far more beneficial in terms of dollars spent on health, number of animals saved, and far less of a carbon footprint.

Dr. Melanie Joy, social psychologist and author of Why We Love Dogs, Eat Pigs and Wear Cows says that accepting animals as a source of food requires us to numb our feelings, distort our thinking and act against our fundamental beliefs of right and wrong. People all over the planet are engaging in this type of behavior, which is completely contrary to humanity's intrinsic values, and it's not because our ancestors did it. Humans, in fact, aren't born violent. We learn it.

Anyone could choose to opt out of this behavior, except that they don't even realize that it might be irrational or destructive. Heck, they don't even know they have a choice in the matter. The irrationality and destruction of this simple behavior is practically invisible.

Understanding how we arrived at eating animals will aid in how we perceive the people around us while moving forward in our journey toward rejecting the status quo. Virtually everyone who grew up eating animals, dairy, and eggs since the turn of the century starts down this path of indoctrination without ever thinking about it critically. Knowing how we arrived at these adopted beliefs dictate how we understand and involve ourselves in the world.

And if we are already keeping animals, eggs, and milk off of our plate, it can help us determine better ways of approaching topics about health, the environment, and the animals when we sympathize with where someone else's mindset may be today.

How did we get here?

I'm the eldest of my siblings. I proudly had a hand in raising and setting an example for my little sister and my baby brother. And, because I was fifteen years old when my brother was born, I can recall as a baby how he emulated everything my sister and I would do (or at least he would attempt to). When we would clap our hands together, so would he. When we would stick out our tongues and make a funny "pffffft" sound, he would too. We always celebrated and gave him praise for following along, and we felt like such great teachers when he complied. And, we may have seemed less enthused with him as soon as he was too tired of following along, or his attention focused on something other than what we were doing. But, after enough encouragement, he always ended up back on track following along with our entertaining shenanigans. Was my baby brother seeking our approval through emulation? Or was he simply playing 'monkey see, monkey do' to improve his own motor skills?

Then, when I was eighteen and in Orlando, I attended a Catholic Mass delivered in Latin with a Catholic friend. I didn't know anything about Catholicism or the functions of a mass, but I found myself looking for social queues from the participants around me so I could follow along with the genuflecting, kneeling, standing and making the sign of the cross from my forehead to my chest, then left shoulder to right shoulder. I had only seen Baptist and non-denominational Christian services before, so the Latin Mass felt like I was taking an aerobics class in a foreign country where I didn't know the language. I was always in anticipation of the next move. I realized that even though I didn't understand what any of it meant, I felt this natural compulsion to fit in and not draw any unwanted attention to myself.

These examples give us clues as to why we have followed the status quo for so long, never knowing if it was truly meant to be our path or the core of who we are. Can you think of examples in your life where you have trusted the actions of others and emulated what they did? It doesn't have to have a negative outcome. I first learned how to put on makeup by watching my mom, and I learned how to start up a business from observing and learning from others who have done it. I learned to eat the way I ate because that's what my parents fed me ever since I was weaned. And it was socially validated as normal as I got older, giving me no cause for concern.

Social psychologists have conducted numerous controlled studies to determine what influences us to conform in such an automatic fashion without critically thinking for ourselves. The general consensus is that we have a fear of being kicked out of our tribe for being different than everyone else.

So when we grow up in a culture that justifies the use and slaughter of animals as food and other commodities, we internalize that this is a normal, natural and necessary behavior. And when we observe our society all around us acting in accordance with this invisible belief, we can easily become susceptible to the billion-dollar marketing campaign messages from the meat, dairy and egg industries whose main agenda is to sell more products and increase profits.

We get entangled in the animal agriculture industry agenda of economic consumerism because we like the taste of the finished animal products, never stopping to think that the majority of us would never voluntarily witness those very animals being massacred in a slaughterhouse.

Furthermore, when the animal agriculture industry convinced our government officials by any means necessary that these animal products are necessary for human health, well, you get an idea of how we ended up in a predicament where animal foods are being subsidized so they can be sold cheaply while fresh organic fruits and vegetables are barely affordable to many members of the working class.

What's dangerous is that it has become a global epidemic for other countries to keep up with the American Jones's. You can grab a cheeseburger or bucket of fried chicken just about anywhere in the world now, and the indigenous people of these countries find it just as addictive as America designed it to be, according to their growing waistlines and plummeting health over the past few decades. Many foreigners around the world see meat-eating as a symbol of wealth. Seems like we should be setting a much better example by now.

We learn how to live by observing how others live. By the time we are old enough to reason, our food habits and preferences have already been ingrained, so there's nothing left to question on the subject of morality until a conflict of our values is triggered - such as in a book or film that depicts the violence towards animals that is caused each time we buy a cheeseburger.

We are even further removed from animal sensitivity as we adopt violence against animals in our everyday language, much like the violent idioms born from many forms of bigotry in our American slang. For instance, "bleeding like a stuck pig," "kill two birds with one stone," "beating a dead horse," "be the human guinea pig," "more than one way to skin a cat," "grab the bull by the horns," and "like a chicken with its head cut off."

We trust in the beliefs and traditions we follow because that's what was already in place before we arrived. Anything that does not align with the traditions we have learned is viewed as weird, abnormal, or *gasp* extreme. Those people who rebel on the other side of our definition of "normal" are either ignored, ridiculed or ostracized. Meanwhile, the conformist rarely stops to think that perhaps it would be worth their time to hear the rebel out.

How many times throughout history have we held a belief that was adopted by the masses that was unjust or didn't make logical sense, yet we created massive violence in its name? Genocide. Slavery. Execution, like beheading and burning at the stake. And gender, racial, religious, cultural and sexual discrimination - all forms of bigotry that we continue as a society to follow the needle of our moral compass and raise a collective conscious tolerance for. Only humans act from a belief system rather than just instincts, even if what we believe isn't necessarily what's right. We are a species that puts morality in high regard, but we can be blinded to what is moral and just if we don't stop to question *why* we do what we do.

Not that long ago, we've used electroshock therapy and lobotomies to "fix" mental illness, depression, homosexuality and chronic pain. It used to be tolerated for periods of time throughout American history for the dominant sect of society to prevent women from equal rights, to label people with special needs a "retard," and a black person a "nigger" until society fully understood the violence and oppression our language perpetuated because of rebels who stood up and changed the minds and hearts of many. And today in many corners of the world, society is still learning social acceptance among the gay, lesbian and transgender communities as we continue to work out the kinks with the pervasiveness of heterosexual supremacy.

The good news is we are on an upward trajectory of treating all humans as we want to be treated - with dignity, respect and kindness, and with the right to the same freedoms as everyone in the majority. As children are raised to see a "human race" with a variety of cultural differences rather than extracting and punishing the minority, and that all people have unique gifts, preferences and challenges, then so too can we begin to show our children how to respect the planet and all the creatures in which we share it with.

Our misshapen belief patterns about ourselves as humans throughout history are parallel to the most overlooked form of exploitation in modern culture called *speciesism*.

Speciesism is defined as the assumption of human superiority which leads to the exploitation of animals. The majority of our human culture clings to a perceived belief that humankind holds superiority over all other living things and beings. And just like the other forms of perceived superiority that we just discussed, speciesism has been cleverly masked by the operations that profit from it.

I believe that once we, the collective human race, begin to understand why and how we got to this place in time where the corrupt pleasure of speciesism thrives, and we use our collective voice to bring about justice for oppressed animal victims, we can be truly free in our minds and hearts. Their freedom is bound to our freedom, for we are all Earth's creatures. And we desire to express the goodness of our humanity, even when it's tough.

Are we psychopaths?

I'm willing to bet that most of the people you know probably think that eating animals is normal, healthy, and necessary. I'm also willing to bet it is their impression that only vegans and vegetarians follow a belief system when it comes to consuming food.

I'm going to burst that bubble, and explain why vegans and vegetarians who used to eat animals *unlearned* the persistent *belief* system of our human culture in eating the flesh and by-products of animals.

It is widely accepted today that sentient animals are conscious beings who feel and exhibit a wide array of emotions including love, joy, happiness, pleasure, empathy, fear, anger, sadness and intense grief. They are capable of holding memories, building relationships, and discriminating between what is safe and what is a threat. Sentient animals, regardless of the species, also decipher physical sensations. Such as when a gentle touch feels good and safe to them, or a hard hit to their bodies and tear of their flesh feels physically painful and a threat to their survival.

Just think of the animals you have come to observe through your life, whether they were your own pets or someone else's that you knew. Take the family dog or cat, for example. Ever accidentally step on their foot or tail and then feel remorse for your mistake because it hurt them? Ever see them cower at a thunderstorm, fireworks, or the raised arm of someone who has hit them? Snuggle in comfort with you or their littermates and purr in contentment, or roll over for oh-so-good belly rubs? Or whined when you left the house because they were distraught to see you go? Whimper and twitch while they're sleeping as you wonder if they are having a good dream or a bad one? And, finally, lovingly clean, feed, and protect their litter of youngins?

Our beloved domestic dogs and cats and with their individual quirks and characteristics also show us that, just like other sentient animals, including the mammals, fowl and marine life we raise as food, they are individuals. While we think of a herd of cows, a group of pigs, or a flock of chickens as a collective with no individuality, the reality is that each of them is an individual with his or her own quirks, demeanor, thoughts and personality.

As humans, we share the same structures and neuro-chemicals of the brain with nonhuman animals, all of which are important in processing and expressing what we are feeling. Therefore, it's not just us and our pets, but every animal, and everyone.

We know cows, chickens, turkeys, ducks, pigs and other farmed animals are individuals on some level, and most of us actually care about the well-being of them, even if we ourselves are not inclined to ever live the lifestyle of a vegan. We want them to live free from harm, and do whatever it is they do in their natural environment. And most of us are appalled and horrified when we hear about or see an animal being treated cruelly or killed unjustly.

Think of the public outcry for moral justification over puppy mills, animal poaching, and instances like the Cincinnati Zoo gorilla named Harambe who was not tranquilized, but killed because of someone's momentary fear after a 3-year old boy fell into the gorilla habitat. Based on the public's response to such "injustices," clearly people care about the lives of animals as much as other people.

We will even go to great measures to protect ourselves from seeing any horrific acts of violence toward animals, and psychologists even classify any person who willingly inflicts pain upon any animal as a *psychopath*.

We even possess the wisdom to teach our children to be nice to animals. We watch as children's eyes light up at the excitement of being in the presence of them. We say "aww" when a small child plays with and nuzzles up to an animal. And most of us have even cared on some level about an animal in our own life.

Have you ever felt warm and fuzzy at the sight of cute baby piglets and newborn chicks just as much as when you see puppies and kittens? Have you ever felt disgusted to learn dogs and cats are raised for meat in some parts of the world, and pondered why they are granted love and a soft bed to sleep on here in our part of the world? Do you ever feel a moral outrage of the torture and pointless slaughter of dolphins in the watery coves of Japan because they are seen as competition for the fishing industries' profit?

Why do we advocate for the pain, suffering and killing of living, sentient beings when it is nowhere near necessary for our own survival today? Do we even know we are advocating such things every time we buy food that contains animal products? Why do most people go through life never asking these kind of questions and or seeking their rational answers? I used to believe it's because that's "just the way it is." But is it really a psychopathic tendency that we allow to continue because it's considered normal, natural, and necessary?

The 4-H Youth Livestock Program and the FFA Supervised Agricultural Experience are apprenticeship programs where young kids purchase young animals, care for them for a period of time, and then sell them at auction for slaughter. This is where socialization meets learned desensitization.

Among the many good and well-meaning goals for the kids that parents and these young farmer programs hope to instill, such as the value of hard work and overcoming challenges, the unnerving skill taught is the practice of detachment from the animals who are in these children's care for the purpose of exploitation. Many of these kids when interviewed after selling their animal acknowledge how difficult it can be to detach from their emotions when they've had a chance to know the animals in their care. And the motivation for the young farmers? Not only is it a cultural tradition that the young people are raised into, but also to earn the most money possible for their college fund at the expense of the auctioned animal's life.

"I was a staunch meat, dairy, egg and honey eater from as far back as I can remember. I wore leather, wool, silk and used other products derived from the bodies of animals. I used products involving animal testing and containing animal secretions. I enjoyed entertainment that involved the use of animals. Essentially, I did what it seemed everyone around me did – the oppressive things society taught me were acceptable – and I did them without a second thought.

I consumed every type of animal flesh that came my way, never once stopping to consider what the consequences of my blind consumption were to my health, the health of the planet and – least of all but *most importantly* – the freedom and lives of the animals I was eating. They were already dead, so I had no part to play in any of that...right?

In 2004 I watched Peaceable Kingdom, a beautiful documentary that gently challenged me to examine my beliefs about non-human animals and I became aware in 70 minutes of what I'd been blind to my entire life: I was complicit in a well-hidden, cruelly concealed global atrocity taking the lives of billions of vulnerable sentient non-human individuals every year. At the end of the film, I sat crying and muttering, "I had no idea... I had no idea...", desperately wondering how I could stop supporting this nightmare. The answer was simple – start living vegan. I began living vegan that moment. It's the best decision I've ever made."

Keith Berger - Boca Raton, FL

We are accustomed to defending our beliefs, and we unconsciously seek validation that what we believe is true. And once we learn the truth about how we arrived to believing that using animals unjustly and unfairly for personal gain is normal or necessary, we no longer need to succumb to the justifications that have kept this system going.

The good news is that simply becoming aware of the beliefs around our dominion over animals in which we have become indoctrinated actually enables us to reclaim our ability to make rational choices. Recognizing the disconnect allows us to make choices according to our value of reverence for the innocent and aids our vision for creating a less violent world.

No matter how you slice it, taking the livelihood, and life, from any being for the purpose of one's own self-interest is an act of violence. Whether we conduct the act of violence with our own hands, or we indirectly have the blood on our hands due to the action of simply paying for it to be done, we are responsible for the persisting violence against animals that want nothing more from us than their freedom. Therefore, we also possess the power to stop it and change our future story to a more just and compassionate one.

Taking back our minds from the old traditions and clever marketers, and thinking critically before we choose what we consume is what eating like you give a damn is all about. Meat, dairy, and egg consumption belongs to the past. Freedom, compassion, and vitality belongs to today.

3

This is Eating
Like You Give a Damn

*"It always seems to me that man was not born to be a
carnivore. Nothing will benefit health and increase the
chances for survival of life on Earth as the evolution to a
vegetarian diet." Albert Einstein*

Eating like you give a damn means choosing compassionately as much as possible in the face of old habits and
traditions involving meat, dairy and eggs, as well as promoting a healthy lifestyle in order to be a kickass advocate.

While the primary motivation to choosing a "vegan" or
"plant-based" path varies depending on the individual, there
are major beneficial secondary outcomes to both since meat,
dairy and eggs are off the table.

However, simply eating a plant-based diet is not the same as being vegan. Just as the term "vegan" is not synonymous with a healthy diet. On the surface, they can look the same. Both promote a diet of grains, legumes, nuts, seeds, vegetables and fruit and also the elimination of animal products including meat, fish, eggs, dairy, gelatin and other animal byproducts from one's diet. So, it's easy to confuse the two based on what is not consumed.

But here is the main difference....

A whole foods plant-based lifestyle is a committed stance towards one's health through nutrition. However, a vegan lifestyle is a committed stance against cruelty towards, unnecessary use of, and exploitation of all animals.

Sometimes a person who is concerned primarily with their health will watch a film like What the Health or Forks Over Knives, and after watching the film, this person may now declare that they are going to take a committed stance in favor of their health and exclude animal flesh and by-products from their diet to be...vegan.

The confusion might come from the fact that today we hear the term "vegan diet" tossed around, which directs our minds to focus on the foods that aren't consumed rather than the intentional avoidance of all acts of animal cruelty. So while this well-intentioned person adopts the term "vegan," it would be more appropriate to refer to their lifestyle as "plant-based" when describing their commitment to their healthy diet.

But what's unique is that I've seen many people go plant-based for their health, and then later identify as vegan once they've witnessed the exploitation and violence towards animals in the name of consumer goods and entertainment. Which means that in addition to eating healthy whole foods plant-based and no animal products, they look for specifically for cruelty-free and vegan friendly products, and they no longer purchase leather goods, or visit zoos, rodeos and circuses. While this can seem restrictive or limiting to the average person who isn't yet open to change, it is actually very empowering. And my intention is for you to understand why this is empowering by the end of this book.

Here is further explanation based on my experience and understanding of the popular terms "plant-based," "whole foods plant-based," and "vegan," as they are all popular terms used interchangeably across many media platforms:

Plant-based = a diet that is mostly plant-dominant and motivated by causing less harm to animals and the planet while lowering the chance of deadly diet-induced illness. This diet is not always plant-exclusive, as some concessions for eating animal products are occasionally made out of convenience, tradition, perceived necessity, or habit. The term plant-based describes a person who is ethically and healthfully aware of the benefits to being vegan, but their commitment to abstaining from all forms of animal products is either growing stronger as they are learning to be more aware, or they find that being mostly plant-based creates the conscious comfort they are looking for. Those living a plant-based lifestyle can closely resemble a reducetarian, but not necessarily an abolitionist. Those ascribing to a plant-based diet also may or may not let their concern for animal exploitation and the Earth's resources cross over into other purchasing habits, such as clothing, household products and personal care products.

Whole Food Plant-Based = (WFPB) this diet is plant-exclusive, and the primary motivation of this abolitionist approach is for personal longevity by avoiding all diet-induced illness. It is self-motivated, and based strictly on scientific, testimonial and personal evidence of disease reversal, prevention and overall improvement to health. The term WFPB was coined by Dr. T. Colin

Campbell after the conclusion of the largest and longest study performed on human nutrition to date called The China Study. WFPB dieters acknowledge the benefits to the planet and animals, however it is not the primary motivation for choosing to adopt this lifestyle. This diet avoids processed oil, white flour and white sugar, and seeks to nearly eliminate the consumption of processed food. There is crossover to health promoting labels of food and other products such as organic, non GMO, local, etc. And those who tend to identify as WFPB for health might also be empathetic to the plight of animals and the planet, or not empathetic at all.

Vegan = this term was coined by English animal rights advocate, Donald Watson, in 1944. This is a plant-exclusive diet and lifestyle which is motivated by consciously avoiding, as much as possible, any use, cruelty and exploitation of all animals within as well as outside of the daily diet. The primary motivation of this abolitionist approach is to exclude all participation of harm towards animals and/or the planet. The vegan diet acknowledges the benefit to the prevention of deadly illness caused by the consumption of animal products. Depending on the individual, the vegan diet does allow processed vegan foods as well as fatty, sugary treats. And when asked about diet, they are typically first vegan for ethical reasons, and then plant-based for health. This is a path of moral consistency where there is crossover to cruelty-free brands that extend outside of diet, such as clothing, household products and personal care products. Vegans fall anywhere on the plant-exclusive spectrum from WFPB to junk food dominant.

Some people believe "vegan" food is different from "normal" food, so if it's labeled "vegan" it must be associated with rigidity or deprivation of what's "normal" or "good." But in reality, *everyone* eats vegan food. So, the moment you reject animal products because of your stance against the injustice and desire for transparency within our food system, it's easy to simply double or triple up on the fruits, vegetables, beans, nuts, seeds, spaghetti, oatmeal, rice, grits, peanut butter and jelly sandwiches, and the many other foods not derived from animals that you've always eaten until you learn about all the new vegan-friendly foods in your grocery store and various restaurants.

You've always eaten "normal" food that is also "vegan," and it's available virtually everywhere. The challenge many people face is reducing and eliminating the animal-based foods they've been used to simply because they didn't realize just how much they consume until they started paying attention.

Is it healthy?

Some people who choose to eat plant-exclusive are unconcerned with their health and therefore don't take the time to research a healthy way of eating, and it's usually by choice. They may eat a diet of predominantly processed vegan foods that mirror the meat and dairy based diet they grew up eating. For example, a bowl of cereal and cup of coffee with nut milk and a vegan donut for breakfast; vegan grilled cheese on white bread and vegan buttery spread alongside vegan jerky, potato chips and a coke for lunch; vegan chik'n patty sandwich with egg-free mayo and bbq sauce on a sesame bun, French fries and a beer for dinner; and Oreos atop vegan ice cream for dessert.

While it is seen as admirable by many vegans for someone to display that comfort foods can still be enjoyed because there is a vegan version of just about everything at your local grocery store these days, Dr. Michael Greger, author of How

Not To Die, warns vegans to resist getting stuck here during their transition from animal-based foods to a vegan lifestyle.

Diet-induced illness can affect vegans and other plant-exclusive dieters just as much as meat and dairy eaters. And while the jury is still out on the long term effects of eating exclusively vegan processed junk foods, any diet regularly void of the nutrition derived from eating whole plant foods can leave the body susceptible to illness and lethargy.

Most vegans are truly concerned about the exploitation of animals. Therefore, those who are advocates of a healthy lifestyle implore "junk food vegans" to incorporate more nutrient dense plant foods into their repertoire to avoid illness, like dark greens, berries, and mushrooms. Because, we've all met that one person who said "My friend so-and-so was vegan and got really sick, but now they eat fish and are feeling better."

Vegan health professionals know there's more to that story and know better than to believe that the animal flesh is what miraculously healed the sick vegan. The presence of certain nutrients in the fish is the likely reason for feeling better. Yet the "junk food vegan" didn't learn that those same nutrients are also found in various plant foods, and therefore their plant-exclusive diet could use some fine tuning. According to physician and educator Dr. Michael Klaper, after analyzing the vegan diets of patients who complain of not feeling well, he says "iodine deficiency is one of the really common causes of vegans failing to thrive."

Which is why it's important for vegans to be health conscious just as much as ethically conscious and eat a plant-exclusive diet rich in various colors of the rainbow, supplemented with vitamin B12, and foods rich in nutrients such as iodine in sea vegetables and omega-3 fatty acids in ground flax and chia seeds, and get a daily dose of vitamin D3 from sunshine. More on this as well as what to eat for optimal health in chapter 7.

Vegans often feel the pressures of being under a microscope, so better to look and feel your very best while being "the change you wish to see in the world (M.K. Ghandi)" in order to effectively convince the people around us to make conscious choices about their purchasing and eating habits. If you're not healthy, they aren't listening.

Sometimes I meet people who discuss their diet with me when finding out that teach about and eat a plant-exclusive diet, and know that they themselves are in poor health and facing their own mortality because they don't like fruits or vegetables. If they are meat-centric, they tell me they are a meat and potatoes kind of person. And if they are vegan, they tell me they are the vegan version of a meat and potatoes kind of person.

For the meat-centric individual, I meet them where they are. There's little chance they will force themselves into a whole food plant based lifestyle right away unless they have already suffered a near death experience related to their diet.

Then, we chat about the many different meat, dairy and egg alternatives of the foods they already love. And while plant-based health professionals don't recommend getting stuck there, the shift toward these mock versions of their comfort foods will promote some health benefits in the interim as they learn to adopt more whole plant-based foods over time for total wellness. The key is to utilize these plant-based meat and dairy alternatives as transition foods. And as more whole fruits, vegetables, nuts, seeds, grains and legumes are adopted regularly, then those alternatives will become more of an occasional treat.

Similarly, when the vegan concerned for their health says they eat the vegan version of a meat and potatoes diet with little to no fruits and veggies, I commend them on the potatoes first, and then I recommend starting the day with a simple smoothie. Many people like the chain Tropical Smoothie, so I tell them to think of their favorite go-to smoothie flavor and mimic that at home, and use little to no sweetener, if possible. Then, over time start introducing power foods like dark greens and flaxseeds to ramp up the nutrition wattage. Once the habit has been created and it is now a daily ritual to begin the day with a smoothie, that becomes the gateway food that leads even the most dedicated junk food connoisseur to greener and healthier pastures.

If you're ready to see what a plant-exclusive diet looks like, visit www.eatinglikeyougiveadamn.com/guide to download your free copy of the Endless Plant-Based Food Guide. It contains the latest omnivore-approved meat, dairy, and egg replacements you can find in your local grocery store, healthy whole food recommendations, and a customizable menu chock full of plant-based foods and a variety of flavors so your vegan meals are never bland or boring.

You're probably wondering now about the "othertarians" that fall under similar categories, like pescatarian, vegetarian, flexitarian and reducetarian. Why is all the buzz today just on vegan and plant-based?

Documentaries, social media and scientific literature promoting a healthy plant-exclusive diet have taken the westernized world by storm. It is no surprise that people find today that if they are to make a dietary improvement, whether on the grounds of health or ethics, vegan and whole food plant-based are the two dominant paths for the knowledgeable and the committed. However, for many around the world, varying degrees of vegetarianism are still practiced.

The term vegetarian came about in the mid-1800's, but the voluntary abstinence from consuming animal flesh was recorded as early as the 6th century BCE and better known as the Pythagorean diet, after the famous Greek philosopher and religious leader Pythagoras.

Vegetarian is a term that describes a diet for people who don't want animals killed for their meals for ethical or religious reasons, or perhaps, simply grossed out by animal flesh.

Vegetarians typically consume eggs and dairy products while being largely unaware of the health and ethical implications of those foods. The largest population of vegetarians in the world are found throughout India, with 30% of its people abstaining from all animal flesh.

Some who flash the vegetarian badge may not always abstain from animal flesh either, making them more flexitarian, reducetarian, or even pescetarian (if fish is on the menu). I know this because I was one of them for a period of time. I described myself as vegetarian when I still included seafood in my diet a few times a month because I didn't critically identify that fish and other sea creatures were not in fact *vegetables*.

"When one of my friends told me "Fred, no one in the world ever proved that meat is necessary in the human diet. That being said, the only reason we do, is for the taste. And that reason is not big enough for me to continue eating it." Well, it wasn't either for me, so 2 weeks after, I was officially vegan. I used to eat steak or other red meat every single day. Never in my life would I have believed that when I now see a bag of kale at the grocery store, I would be so happy! I started by being really discreet about being vegan, but now I think that the world is super open to learning a new way to do things and new way of living their life. I will continue to encourage people to eat more plants, inspiring new vegans, one at a time."

Frederic Tristan - Montreal, Quebec

Is it all or nothing?

Being a rebel for compassion and making more ethical choices is not about purity. It's about progress. And I'm not just talking about our progress at home. But also the incremental progress we make together as a society towards creating demand in the marketplace for more cruelty-free consumer goods. As we are witnessing in various global statistics, such as those that you'll find listed in Chapter 8, when ethical consumerism goes up, the demand for meat, dairy and eggs goes down. Also, more money is invested by mammoth food companies for the creation of innovative vegan foods that replace the ones made with animal ingredients. Now ain't that a beaut?!

While it's true that many people identify strongly with their vegan lifestyle, making ethical choices is ultimately about achieving impact. Do as much as you possibly can to reduce animal product consumption. As vegan advocate and author Colleen Patrick-Goudreau says, "Don't do nothing because you can't do everything. Do something. Anything."

Most vegans were once omnivores, and while some can quit "cold turkey," not everyone can change their diet overnight. What matters most is to be aware and take responsibility to move in the right direction. Some people find it easier to make radical changes, while others take a more progressive path. Aim high, but don't let the unrealistic image of perfection be the enemy of the greater good.

Keep in mind that chickens kept in cages or crowded enclosures for their flesh and eggs suffer greatly, and because they are small animals, many individuals are needed to feed a family over the course of days, weeks, months and years. So replacing chickens and eggs with a healthy plant-based alternative for those meals, or with vegan mock products like Vegan Egg by Follow Your Heart, or Beyond Chicken Strips by Beyond Meat, could be a great place to begin if you haven't already.

Similarly, every fish caught is a whole animal, as well as numerous "by-catch" animals, that all suffered for that one meal. Times that by the number of times you are used to consuming fish products and you can see how much of an impact you have when you begin to swap those out with animal-free foods, like Fish Free Tuna by Good Catch, or Crabless Cakes by Gardein.

Because of your interest in this book, chances are that you are aware of the immense suffering of pigs, dairy cows, beef cows and other animals commonly used for food. Perhaps you have already begun to reduce or have eliminated these from your meal plans. Kudos, fellow rebel!

Aside from combating injustice and to cruelty to animals, you will be contributing to your own health while combating injustice for future generations by reducing your own contribution to climate change and environmental degradation. Who knew that being a rebel against the status quo could be so globally and enduringly impactful?

4

Start with Your "Big Why"

"I do not see any reason why animals should be slaughtered to serve as human diet when there are so many substitutes. Life is as dear to a mute creature as it is to a man. Just as one wants happiness and fears pain, just as one wants to live and not to die, so do other creatures." The Dalai Lama XIV

Plant-based eating may not be entirely mainstream yet. However, it's becoming more and more accepted every day, and this trend is having far-reaching impacts. Everyone from professional athletes and celebrities to entire companies like Google and countries as big as China are supporting the movement to eat more plant-based foods.

But people don't actively seek out a reason for cutting back on or eliminating animal products. Wrapped in the comfort of our own traditions, we don't know what we don't know. And when we do know it and we are moved emotionally by it, then we are empowered to do something about it.

When we have a big enough "why" for changing something that has otherwise been comfortable, we will accept any "how." It's important to understand that the Big Why, or reason for choosing to follow a plant-exclusive lifestyle, is motivated by meaning, purpose and emotion. And while many people are inclined to think that willpower is the key to making consistent choices, it's your *emotion* that drives your *behavior.* Not willpower.

Some people have experienced a near death experience, or lost a loved one to a health condition brought on by poor dietary and lifestyle habits. Some people have listened to factory farm workers recount their horrific memories of pigs rubbing against their leg for affection just before inflicting unbearable pain on them as they screamed and fought for their lives. Some people watch a film, attend an event, hear a talk, or receive a warning from their doctor that either tugs on their heart strings or scares the shit out of them, and that becomes their catalyst for change. It's our emotions that either keep us stuck and unwilling to change, or force us to do something different.

So before I can offer up the solution and the steps to live the mission, we first have to start with what's wrong. The following are just some of the facts that have recently elevated a movement whose mission began on ethical grounds to eradicate all forms of exploitation and cruelty to animals. And today, this mission has evolved into 3 main pillars of the collective movement toward plant-based eating that affect more than just the well-being of animals, but all of us humans as well. The 3 pillars are health, animals, and the environment. And because each one is just as intertwined with the outcomes of another, I call this the vegan trifecta.

The Trifecta

For Our Health:

Below are just some of the researched and proven benefits published throughout various medical and nutrition journals for adopting a wholesome vegan diet - rich in fiber, phytonutrients, antioxidants, vitamins and minerals, and free of cholesterol; low in calories and saturated fat. They include:

a. Quick and sustainable fat loss

b. Improved cholesterol, blood pressure and triglycerides

c. Lowered risk of coronary heart disease

d. Improved insulin function while managing and even reversing Type 2 diabetes

e. Lowered risk of developing certain types of cancer: such as breast, ovarian and prostate cancer, as well as colorectal cancer

f. Increased fertility and balance of hormones

g. Clear acne and eczema

h. Ease arthritis pain, build strong bones, improve gut, liver and bowel health

i. Create a more alkaline environment while reducing risk of kidney stones

j. And may help prevent Alzheimer's and other forms of dementia

A vegan diet has been cited as being healthier than diets containing animal products by many studies, both in terms of disease prevention and treatment. For instance, one study published in the international, peer-reviewed journal

Nutrients in 2014, which examined the overall diet quality based on different aspects of healthful dietary models, indicated consistently the vegan diet as the most healthy one.

A study performed over 14 years and published in the Journal of Clinical Oncology in 2011 using over 1.1 million people found that cancer feeds on cholesterol to grow. Therefore, a diet free from cholesterol, which is achieved by a whole foods vegan diet, dramatically reduces the risk of developing certain cancers.

The American Dietetic Association has taken the position that "appropriately planned vegetarian diets, including vegan diets, are healthful, nutritionally adequate, and may provide health benefits in the prevention and treatment of certain diseases. Well-planned vegan diets are appropriate for individuals during all stages of the life cycle, including pregnancy, lactation, infancy, childhood, and adolescence, and for athletes."

Besides avoiding cholesterol, saturated fat, high caloric density and carcinogens found in animal products, vegan diets omit the by-products of industrialized animal agriculture such as added growth hormones, as well as hormones naturally present in the animal, most foodborne pathogens, antibiotics and antibiotic resistant bacteria. Conversely, a whole foods vegan diet is higher in fiber, antioxidants, and vitamins and minerals which promote excellent health.

For more information on the health benefits of a whole foods vegan diet, refer to the Resources page in the back of this book.

For the Animals:

There's no way to sugar coat the gross injustices and horrors of producing, raising, and slaughtering billions upon billions of land and sea animals for food, clothing, and other consumer products. Believe me, I've tried. All I can offer are some of the cold hard facts and a nudge to watch a documentary film that will bring these well hidden mysteries to light, such as Peaceable Kingdom, Earthlings, and Food, Inc. I have included a comprehensive list of where to find helpful media and resources such as these in the back of this book.

It takes courage to bear witness to the common animal agriculture practices that inflict a kind of suffering most people could never imagine in their own minds. Nothing else quite illustrates the reality that these individuals experience once we bring them into this world and then take them out of it just to fatten someone's wallet. The good news is that you can decide to remove yourself from this system and be perfectly healthy by choosing a plant-exclusive diet, and I'll show you throughout this book just how easily it can be done.

Over *56 billion* farmed animals are slaughtered each year by humans for food. That comes out to over 153 million animals killed around the world for food each day. This figure does not include sea creatures whose deaths are so great they are measured in *tonnes*. Each of the chickens, cows, pigs, turkeys, ducks, fish, and others - including bycatch and predatory animals - who are killed for human use are sentient beings with complex central nervous systems which allow them to feel pain and to suffer.

In addition to the act of slaughter which inherently causes a great deal of unnecessary pain, fear, and suffering, the methods by which animals are bred, raised, confined, and transported are, by any reasonable definition, inhumane. Young animals are often ripped away from their mothers moments after birth, unhealthy animals are pushed by bulldozers into trash heaps while in agony, and animals often die from unbearable conditions during long, cramped transports to other farms and slaughterhouses.

The meat, dairy, egg, veal, wool, down and leather industries are all closely connected and interdependent. Consuming dairy and eggs contributes directly to the meat industries.

From male chicks being ground up or suffocated alive by the egg industry, to the leather industry being directly funded by meat, to the male calves of dairy cows being used for veal - it is impossible to consume non-meat animal by-products, like dairy, eggs and gelatin, without benefiting the meat industries and causing animal suffering.

Mahatma Gandhi, a lifelong vegetarian and freedom fighter, wrote in his autobiography, "To my mind, the life of a lamb is no less precious than that of a human being. I should be unwilling to take the life of a lamb for the sake of the human body. I hold that, the more helpless a creature, the more entitled it is to protection by man from the cruelty of man."

If you've ever envisioned Old MacDonald's happy farm of cows, pigs, horses, chickens, ducks and goats grazing in the pasture until old age, and then being "humanely stunned" before they go blissfully to farm animal heaven like I did... well, not only is this not their reality, but I'm willing to bet their day-to-day life at a factory farm is far worse than you could ever imagine.

I believe there is a way for us to have a symbiotic relationship with farmed animals. As the human population demands less of their meat and by-products, farmers artificially inseminate less of them over time until it is unsustainable for them to keep producing them unnaturally at all. And as the animal population decreases due to less demand, farmers can humanely reenlist what benevolent homesteaders had been doing for centuries to grow organic crops. Cows, goats, and pigs tend to the aeration and mowing of the land, and fowl keep the parasites like mosquitos and fleas at bay - all without the need for force as this is what their instincts are to do naturally. Farmers reciprocate the favor by supplying shelter, food, and safety from natural predators, thereby allowing farm animals a safe environment to form bonds and experience love, just like our domesticated companion animals at home. There's no need to kill them and eat their bodies or by-products on grounds of health as well as environmental factors. Which brings me to the final pillar of the vegan trifecta...

For the Environment:

As we are currently spiraling out of control with catastrophic impacts on our environment caused by factory farming, I implore you to imagine what our environment must have been like before the following statistics became our reality.

A 2010 United Nations report said that a global shift towards a vegan diet is vital to save the world from hunger, fuel poverty, and the worst impacts of climate change.

Animal agriculture is environmentally unsustainable. From the widespread contamination of drinking water supplies in North Carolina by hog manure runoff to the the rise of drug-resistant pathogens as the result of feeding antibiotics to chickens on factory farms.

Producing meat, dairy, eggs, leather, wool, and so forth cycles finite resources through animals to achieve a net loss of resources. The United Nations Commission on Sustainable Development reported that it takes up to 7,000 liters of water to produce 100 grams of beef in developing countries, while it takes just 550 liters of water to produce enough flour for one loaf of bread.

Further, a global assessment of the water footprint of farm animal products was published in the academic journal Ecosystems in 2012 and it concluded that the water footprint of any animal product is larger than the water footprint of crop products with equivalent nutritional value. Twenty-nine percent of the total water footprint of the agricultural sector in the world is related to the production of animal products, with the average water footprint per calorie for beef found to be 20 times larger than for cereals and starchy roots, and the water footprint per gram of protein for milk, eggs, and chicken meat found to be 1.5 times larger than for legumes, for example.

In terms of land use, livestock now covers 45 percent of the earth's entire land surface. And, 33 percent of the global arable land used to produce feed for livestock is desertified, meaning the land is now too dry or barren to support vegetation. Further, animal consumption is a major driver of deforestation, with 91 percent of Amazon rainforest destruction caused by animal agriculture.

With regards to global climate change, one of the most pressing environmental issues of our time, experts cite that livestock and their by-products account for 51 percent of greenhouse gas emissions, which is far more than all methods of transportation by car, train, plane, and boat *combined*.

In addition to unsustainable resource consumption and contribution to global climate change, animal agriculture serves as a major source of air, water, and soil pollution. According to the EPA, "A single dairy cow produces about 120 pounds of wet manure per day, which is equivalent to the waste produced by 20-40 people." Additionally, the EPA reports that the waste generated by animal agriculture has polluted over 35,000 miles of river in 22 of the United States.

Ground soil is also degraded by nutrients and heavy metals present in animal feed which are inevitably excreted by livestock. When concentrated due to the unsustainable practices of animal agriculture, zinc, copper, chromium, arsenic, cadmium and even lead, build up in the soil and reduce fertility, runoff into water, and end up in the human food supply.

Into our air, factory farms emit harmful gases and particles such as methane and hydrogen sulfide, which can contribute to air quality degradation and harm the health of those living or working nearby.

Even free-range, cage-free, pasture/grass-raised, organic, and local meat, eggs and dairy still require more land, water, fossil fuels, chemicals, and feed inputs and are more polluting than sustainable methods of agriculture such as organic vegetable and fruit production, permaculture, agroforestry, urban gardening, and hydroponics.

When asked why she is a vegan, the primatologist, ethologist, anthropologist, Jane Goodall said, "We now know that intensive meat eating, which is getting more common all around the world, is horribly damaging to the environment, as well as being terribly cruel".

According to environmental scientists, plant-based foods are generally far easier to produce, use less water, and generate a substantially lower environmental footprint than do animal foods. In contrast, the practice of obtaining animal foods for human consumption devastates the environment on many different fronts, and is plainly not sustainable at current and ever-growing demand levels.

For more information about the environmental impacts of animal agriculture, please refer to Resources page in the back of this book.

"Our journey started with a general dislike of the commercial food industry and an interest in living sustainably. We felt that commercial agriculture was producing food that was no longer nutritious or tasteful and that our leaders were failing miserably in containing the environmental impact of our archaic agriculture system.

With this in mind, we decided to buy some land, homestead, raise and slaughter our own meat and grow our own vegetables.

We volunteered for a wildlife rehabilitation organization which would occasionally release native birds and such on our property. One day they asked if we could take in a small pig that had been thrown off a boat and left for dead by its previous owner. We adopted him and began to real ize how sentient he was. He became our best friend and needless to say we gave up pork.

Next, a local rancher asked for help finding an abandoned calf. The mother had broken her hip during birth, wandered off and died and the calf was nowhere to be seen. We searched for two days and just before giving up we spotted him. The rancher asked if we would raise the calf for him and said he would take it back when it was weaned. The rancher did not get his calf back, we quit eating red meat and the calf, Moobee, is a 4-year-old steer that lives with us to this day. He became our dear friend and dare I say an ambassador for his species.

Our process was gradual, but we realized we wanted to save farm animals not eat them or exploit them. We decided to create a farm animal sanctuary where these animals would be given the dignity they deserve. We felt that if we could give a voice to these animals that even a ripple may have an impact.

One day we received a call from Stephanie saying she wanted to visit our farm and meet the animals. She asked if we were vegan, and at this point we were not for we still ate some animal products. Even though we told her we were not vegan she still wanted to come out and visit. I remember that day and the conversation we had was one of compassion for animals and the planet and how we could change things for the better. Her visit completed our path to a cruelty-free diet.

Veganism is not a trend, it is a movement and we are growing. As we grow into a movement our message should be heard at the voting booth where we must put animal rights and the environment at the forefront of our conversations with our leaders and vote people in who realize all lives matter."

Kelly McCormick - Florida Rescue Farm, Duette, FL

Peek Through the Vegan Lens

If you could live healthy and happy without causing violence toward animals, and destruction to our planet, why wouldn't you? It's a strong question, and one that I've asked myself many times over.

During moments when I found myself disconnected from my Big Why because I was in the learning stage; or for convenience, habit, taste, or fear that I would displease my grandma by opting out of eating the pierogi she had seasoned using animal parts; that Big Question helped me to examine my own conscience in order to make the best choice for me in any given situation.

I believe that asking yourself that Big Question when you find it difficult to make compassionate food choices, you will find yourself tapped in and turned on to your Big Why. I think that, then, you will feel quite rebellious and compelled to reject the status quo of eating animals and their by-products.

I first heard about the negative impacts to my health of ingesting chemicals and artificial additives after reading a book called Skinny Bitch, and although I was shocked and angry, it moved me enough to make some adjustments in where I shopped and what foods I bought. And, it made me sad that the majority of people didn't know about the negative impacts on human health from these additives designed by our very own food system. But, to be completely transparent with you, I don't always choose organic and additive-free foods even though I am aware of the consequences. If the food budget is tight or the selection is limited and I have to choose the non-organic produce, or I have a craving for Swedish Fish (Red-40, anyone?), I am known to make concessions. And I feel grateful that at least I'm making an informed and moderated choice that I understand may impact my health in some way.

However, as a committed rebel for compassion today, I don't make concessions for animal products. Period. Why?

Because while I once liked the taste of meat, cheese, eggs, and cream in my coffee, I have the power to stand for what I believe by opting out of those animal derived foods and cause a disruption in the industry. Once I made the *decision* to cut out the last non-vegan foods I held onto as a pescatarian after realizing my money fueled a system that made my heart heavy, it all became easy. I let go of my fears and anxiety around no longer fitting in with my friends and family, no longer knowing what to order when I go out to eat, and not knowing if it was truly good for my health. And guess what? I realized all of that fear and anxiety I held onto was wasted energy. Turns out it's actually cool to be kind. And, of course, it's easy to still enjoy all those same foods I once loved because today there is a vegan version of just about everything.

So, while I value my health and strive to make healthier choices for my physical well-being and longevity, that wasn't what propelled me into making vegan choices. I was more moved by the idea that if I couldn't force a pregnancy on an animal and steal her baby while they cried for each other, and if I couldn't dump newborn baby chicks into a grinder or tie them up alive in a plastic bag, and if I couldn't mutilate animal's body parts without anesthesia or pain care while they writhed and screamed in agony, and if I couldn't destroy delicate ocean habitats and suffocate marine animals, and if I couldn't slit an animal's throat and watch the life drain from their eyes...then I had no business paying for it to be done on my behalf. All of these horrors and more are perpetuated by the mighty dollar, and this was no longer getting my vote.

When I bared witness to what happens to dairy cows, beef cattle, hogs, egg laying hens, lambs, chickens and turkeys, and other animals we consider food, I didn't just see it with my eyes while coddling myself under a blanket of assumed justifications and disbelief. I saw it with my heart, and I felt it in my soul. As a human, I am an animal too, so it wasn't difficult for me to connect to the animal's experience.

I took on those emotions that the animals were experiencing and I watched as though I was seeing it happen through their eyes. I experienced what they must have felt, like the feeling of there being something more to my life that I didn't get to experience because I was unlucky enough to be born on the factory floor with a price tag on my head. I took on the joy of giving birth to my baby and felt the desire to nurture her, feel connected with her and teach her everything I knew. And then I felt the agonizing despair when someone dragged her away from me as I cried out for days, desperate for her to be returned back into my motherly care. I felt the hopelessness that there was nothing I could do to protect my baby and the grief of losing my child as machines were affixed to my tender nipples to rob my body of the nourishment that my body produced for my baby.

I imagined that it was me being electric-prodded down the crowded kill shute while smelling the blood of the victims before me and hearing their wails and screams in the next room while feeling the terror of my impending death. I felt the terror and the desire to fight in order to live, but I could see I was trapped and the force of the humans was so mighty that I had no chance of escape. I saw as though it was me being stunned momentarily and waking in excruciating pain while dangling upside down from one of my legs, and then watching with my own eyes as people with machines hacked away at my body parts, tore the skin right off of my body and pulled my insides apart until I finally bled out.

This became my Big Why because, as you can see, I am empathetic to animal suffering. And seeing an end to that kind of suffering is my driving force to making compassionate choices today.

In today's society, we humanize our companion animals. We get a kick out of giving a human voice to their quirky behaviors. We connect with them in this way on a personal level and find our lives a bit lighter and happier by spending our money to further enrich their life's experience. We buy them food, treats and toys. We take them to the vet when they get sick. We take them on walks even when we don't feel like it. We even let them sleep in our beds and put a wet blanket on our sex lives sometimes. We spare no expense at making them happy because it makes us happy.

We even turn all kinds of animals into loveable characters in story books, cartoons and films. We teach our children that we are to be kind and gentle in the presence of animals, and we coo when they wrap their tiny arms around an animal and love on them. We decorate our children's rooms with stuffed animals and pay special attention not to lose the one they've developed an attachment to. We buy our kids food with their favorite animals on the package and even buy food itself in the shapes of various animals. We take them to a petting farm so they can interact with the real life versions of the cartoon animals they love, and we feel such joy at seeing them happy. All while eating hot dogs topped with chili and cheese and sucking down milkshakes.

So when that humanization and inherent love for animals stops at the end of our fork as we place animal flesh into our mouths, we have to wonder who are the crazy ones, the vegans or everyone else?

Making compassionate choices is not about putting oneself into a self-imposed food prison. It's about arriving to a place of genuine enlightenment about how our actions affect all life. Once we stop flirting with the idea of making vegan choices and actually dig into *why* it's important for us to take responsibility for the health of the bodies we have been given to house our soul, as well as the animals who are negatively impacted, it actually becomes easy to stick to our guns.

For example, just after deciding I was no longer going to eat any animal products, I found myself faced with the temptation of fresh baked cookies when I was working as a bartender in a restaurant. The chef had baked them special for a VIP guest and invited me to have one. It surprised me that I didn't even hesitate to take a bite, and I immediately tried to justify it by thinking to myself "well, I didn't buy it, therefore what's the harm if I didn't personally contribute to the existence of this non-vegan cookie?" And as I chewed and acknowledged just how amazing it tasted, the faces of those who were hurt for the ingredients contained in the cookie flashed in my mind. I thought of the mama cow who cried for her baby calf that was taken away from her just so some of her milk could end up in the chocolate chips...and a helpless male chick who had just hatched into the world was killed, while a female hen lived sick and cramped in a cage too small for her to extend her wings to produce the eggs. Suddenly, that cookie didn't taste so good anymore. I realized in that very moment that nothing tastes as good to me as standing up for the freedom of those animals to live as nature intended, and *not* how humans have intended, which is part of a system that oppresses and harms them for personal gain. Ever since then, when offered something that isn't vegan, I politely decline and look for the opportunity to constructively inform my gifter about why, when appropriate.

Some may reach the conclusion that animal products are no longer good enough for them to consume on ethical grounds after reading just one book, watching just one film, or having just one conversation about their personal contribution to animal suffering because they have an already established connection to their empathy for sentient beings. This may be because they have experienced a personal relationship with a companion animal like dog, cat, or horse over the years and they recognize that the slab of meat on their plate (or the product of an over milked cow or overworked hen) whose well-being is ignored because of the profit margin, may as well have been their own dog, cat, or horse.

Not everyone, however, can make that connection so quickly, or even at all. Others may be in a state of disbelief about animal suffering and require several exposures of bearing witness over time from different sources before something finally clicks. Others are apathetic and chalk it up to yet another crime of humanity without making the connection that one's own purchasing habits make them either a part of the problem or the solution.

Unlike 30 years ago, more people are moving along the path towards becoming vegan for more reasons than just the animals. We now know the catastrophic effects on health and the environment by helping to perpetuate the animal agriculture industry. So, while there are animal sympathizers like myself who find our biggest and most motivating Big Why in helping to end the violence inflicted upon the voiceless, others can be predominantly on the plant-exclusive path because research today shows us how a whole foods plant-based diet is arguably one of the healthiest ways for humans to eat. And even more are seeing the profound scientific evidence of the planets destruction caused by animal agribusiness and how one can't really be an environmentalist while purchasing and eating animal-based foods.

While there are challenges and annoyances we encounter as soon as we cross the threshold of our compassionate home and into our non-vegan world, a committed rebel for compassion doesn't feel the chains of restriction. Rather, they are living on purpose and with purpose because they have a Big Why. Rebels for compassion take on a responsibility that requires much of their empathetic energy to set a gentler example of what it means to be human in whatever fashion that suits their natural demeanor, even in the face of the human traits that keep many people out of touch with their very own innate compassion.

Now, we move forward to uncover some action items that will help you along the continuum of being an effective and happy Rebel for Compassion. First order of business is everyone's favorite topic: food!

5

Experiment With Food

"If you change the way you look at things, the things you look at change." Wayne Dyer

I t's tempting to think that the moment you make the decision to live in a plant-based paradise that your transformation into it magically happens overnight. Once the light bulb comes on and you make that compassionate connection, the mindset to live a cruelty-free, eco-friendly or healthy lifestyle becomes the new focus. But how do you really start?

You could, in theory, wake up fully prepared to toss out everything from your refrigerator and cupboard that was produced by using animal derived ingredients, hit the grocery store armed with your Endless Plant-Based Food Guide that you downloaded from eatinglikeyougiveadamn.com/guide, thereby restocking your kitchen with delicious new plant strong foods. And you could, presumably, declare your home as a happy sanctuary away from the products of suffering and destruction that you witness around you every time you leave your house.

However, the reality is that for you it may not be quite that simple. You may stumble quite a bit on your way to joyful Veganville. And, you won't be helping anyone by being an overnight plant strong sensation and reaching total burnout in just a few weeks.

Although people say that they "don't eat a lot of meat, dairy, and eggs," the reality is that one has no idea how much they're consuming until they stop intentionally. To get an idea, start by taking a few minutes to write down what you ate and drank from the last few days (breakfast, lunch, dinner, snacks, drinks). Don't forget to include what you put in your coffee, the spread you put on a sandwich, the cheese you sprinkle on your pasta, or the snack you purchased from the vending machine at your job. This will help you clearly see the incremental changes you should be considering as you start down the path of rebelliously compassionate living. But don't let this drag you down if your list of animal derived ingredients is longer than you thought it might be. Self-awareness is actually very enlightening, and is key to making intentional choices that are in alignment with what you value in life.

Oopsies will happen, and when they do, you might feel a twinge of defeat. Maybe there is a pancake mix you've been buying for the last 15 years, and perhaps you never thought to check the label to see whether there is a milk derived ingredient called whey in the mix. And that sandwich joint near your workplace where you have fallen in love with their vegan burger? You may later find out that the brioche bun they serve it on has butter and eggs in it. It may feel agitating when you discover your efforts of remaining cruelty-free to animals can be derailed, and not by your choice. That's part of the learning curve that makes this a journey.

I've heard people say to me "but animal products are in *everything*, so what's the point in trying?" The point is that to most people who have made a habit of "trying" actually succeed, while those who struggle with the idea of getting started don't understand the true cost of not trying. To those who see difficulty in getting started, animal products are just ingredients. But rebels for compassion know what's at stake if they don't give their best effort in avoiding those products caused by the suffering of animals. And rebels are not willing to compromise on that for their own convenience.

The path to going from zero to fully compassionate living is different for everyone, so it's important to transfer some of that newfound compassion onto yourself as you approach your purchases more cautiously. Remember, it's far better to do a little at a time than to do nothing at all.

And, I'll let you in on a little secret…no vegan is perfect. We still slip up sometimes and say silly things. And, no matter how much kale we eat, the reality is we're all going to die someday. As human beings, we are always a work in progress. But the important thing is to note the progress we make, because in the end, it all adds up in a significant way for more than just ourselves. In the case of progressing towards a rebelliously compassionate lifestyle, the effects reach near and far physically, emotionally, spiritually, locally and globally.

If you are someone who has kicked bad habits in the past and never looked back, like cigarettes, drugs, an overconsumption of alcohol, or maybe you bid adieu to a toxic relationship, then perhaps you are prewired for making a permanent and immediate shift to a compassionately chosen menu.

If you're not skilled in the art of kicking old habits, then start wherever you are today, and make a conscious effort to expand your knowledge and skills as you implement new plant-based foods. And no matter what bumps in the road you hit along the way, always focus on the positive progress you are making.

The stronger your convictions about the various injustices within our food system, the easier it will be to convert, and more importantly, the less you will feel tempted to revert. At the beginning, eating plant-based takes some getting used to, and you may at times feel deprived of foods you are used to enjoying.

But, once you focus on all the variety of plant-based vegan foods that are available to you, there is very little that you will soon be missing. In fact, you may end up finding more pleasure from cooking, using different seasonings, discovering different foods and being creative with new recipes - you'll be cooking your plants off in no time. Heck, you might even become a badass for bringing vegan food to a party that everyone else that isn't vegan raves over!

Start with What's Familiar

The easiest way to glide into plant-based paradise and handle your natural cravings for flavors and textures that are familiar is to take into account each of your next meals and see how you can make them meat-free, dairy-free or egg-free. If you're starting out like I did, I wanted to first veganize the foods I was currently eating before making a complete diet overhaul of food that was foreign to me. So, your mission, should you choose to accept it, is to crowd out the oldies. Here are a few suggestions, each customizable, if you're looking to ease into the transition of a healthy vegan lifestyle:

- Order your next pizza with all veggies and sans cheese. Some places, like Whole Foods, has vegan shredded cheese as a topping for an easy swap if you're itching for it

- Try taco night with Beyond Meat beefy crumbles, or try lentils or black beans in place of the beef. Nix the dairy based cheese in favor of an easy cashew nacho cheese recipe, and try a dollop of Tofutti vegan sour cream (or top with creamy guacamole instead)

- Have spaghetti marinara instead of meat sauce until you find your new favorite vegan pasta recipe

- Order a variety of vegetable sushi rolls without eel sauce, and smuggle in your own homemade spicy mayo made of eggless Just Mayo and Sriracha

- Trade in your cream cheese for a vegan version, like Go Veggie, for your morning bagel. And dairy-free creamer like Califia Farms Better Half for your coffee

- If you're jonesing for ready-made sweets from your local grocer, Ben & Jerry's and So Delicious have dairy-free ice cream in several popular flavors, Oreos are vegan by default, many quality dark chocolate bars are dairy-free, or head to Whole Foods for a plethora of options in their bakery like cakes, cookies and doughnuts

- Turn your beef stroganoff into mushroom stroganoff, and meatloaf into a quinoa-bean loaf. Then whip mashed potatoes with Earth Balance buttery spread and Tofutti vegan sour cream

- Replace the meat in your signature chili recipe with kidney, black or chili beans and add chopped veggies like peppers, zucchini, onions, carrots and corn for more texture and flavor

- Trade the meat in your Asian dishes with tofu, shelled soybeans, cashews or peanuts

- Instead of your usual tuna or chicken salad for sandwiches, pulse drained chickpeas in a food processor and prepare the same way with your new favorite aquafaba mayo recipe. You can also dice Beyond Meat chick'n strips and mix with Just Mayo for mock chicken salad, or Fish Free Tuna by Good Catch with Veganaise for mock tuna salad

- Don't forget fresh fruit and salads. Have apple slices with peanut butter, or make a simple fruit salad. Ditch the dairy cheese and croutons, and swap dairy-laced dressings for a squeeze of lemon to brighten your salads until you find your new favorite vegan dressing.

If at first you become overwhelmed, just focus on how you can veganize your next meal. Eventually, and after one meal at a time, you will find that it gets easier as you go. And before you know it, you will be eating plant-based by habit while also determining what new things you like and don't like.

Start today by focusing on enjoying a menu of items from the plant-based kingdom. Don't worry about the upcoming holiday, what you might eat during your upcoming business trip, or at your friend's wedding in the spring. Don't even worry about what you might be craving during certain ritualistic activities, like movie night or your family trip to the fair. Just think about today, one meal at a time, and plan your next grocery trip accordingly.

Within the plant-based realm, you will find many subcultures. Some are healthier than others, and some seem to duke it out over which reigns as healthiest of all. Some focus on a high density of micronutrients. Some are raw foodists. Some are locavores and keep to local and organic. Some grow their own organic plant fare. Some are quite close to gourmet chefs, and others are not too concerned with such variety or gastronomic pleasure. And some are quite satisfied with living on French fries, soda, and Oreos because their soul is well fed by simply keeping animals off the menu.

Just before I began my journey to making compassionate food choices, I used to watch and follow Rachael Ray's 30-Minute Meals because, as a busy gal, I needed to learn how to get my comfort foods to the table fast. So I began with veganizing familiar comfort foods, and then experimenting with different dessert recipes. Then, I began growing some of my own produce in an aeroponic garden, and learning how to make my plant based diet even healthier without compromising flavor and mouthfeel. And, I still prefer to have my meals ready in 30 minutes or less.

Wherever you find yourself fitting in today, beginning your transition to a plant-strong lifestyle by mirroring how you currently eat will lessen the feeling of being overwhelmed.

And if your goal is to do better than where you are because you want to overcome an illness, shed unwanted weight, or stop feeling like crap all the time, then get in touch with your Big Why and focus on the unprocessed, unpackaged whole foods first (and not vegan grilled cheese and pizza).

Download your free copy of the Endless Plant-Based Food Guide at www.eatinglikeyougiveadamn.com/guide. It contains omnivore approved meat, dairy, and egg replacements, healthy whole food recommendations, and a customizable menu chock full of easy to find plant-based foods and flavors so your vegan meals are never bland or boring. It will be a godsend during your next grocery store trip.

"I was tired of being overweight, tired of feeling like crap and just tired of being and feeling unhealthy in general. I decided my New Year's resolution 2017 would be to change that.

For the first 6 months I focused on eating healthier and losing weight - and it was working! By June I had lost 25 pounds! But, I still felt like crap.

After watching "What The Health" and " Fat, Sick and Nearly Dead" I decided just eating better wasn't enough. I wanted to truly eat and LIVE a healthy life. But...I could never completely give up burgers, pizza, and all my favorite comfort foods...could I? I started by trying to cut out dairy for 2 weeks. And Wow! I felt amazing! And as a bonus, I was able to completely get rid of my acid reflux along with the daily medicine for it!

The plan was to slowly remove one type of item at a time (beef, then chicken and fish, followed by processed foods and oils) but I was enjoying creating new truly healthy recipes and the great way I was feeling so much that I removed EVERYTHING else during week 3! The groups on Facebook have helped tremendously with support and recipes!

The transformation over the last 5 months has been amazing! Not only have I lost an additional 45 pounds but I feel wonderful! My cravings and desires are now for things like roasted vegetables and healthy soups instead of fast food and junk. I feel healthier at almost 46 than I was at 30. For me this is NOT a diet - it's a new - and better way of life!"

Angie Phillips - Salem, OH

Some people report that after eating a meat, dairy, and junk food diet for a long time and suddenly quit, they experienced detox symptoms for several days, like headaches and irritability. Just don't be alarmed thinking that eating a wholesome vegan diet isn't for you. In fact, the detoxing effect should be celebrated! As soon as you get through it and feel like a million bucks afterwards, that is. Everyone has a different experience, and most people I talk to go straight to feeling more energetic after replacing non-vegan foods with clean vegan ones. If your symptoms drag on though, seek the advise of a medical doctor who is well versed in whole foods plant-based nutrition.

Should you experience a setback, don't beat yourself up with regret. Do the best you can with what you've got, and tomorrow begins a new day with a clean slate. As you learn how to navigate challenges with ingredients and vegan food availability, celebrate every success as you grow into a deeper commitment of conscious living.

Here are some tips to help set you up for success and to thwart setbacks.

Tip #1 - Keep meal options in sight. As you replace old animal based or junk food based meals with a healthier vegan version, add it to your "approved meals" list and keep it visible on the fridge (mine is on a magnetic white-board). As you take inventory before your next grocery trip, it will save you time just to glance at your fridge to jog your memory of meals you already like versus thumbing through cookbooks and websites.

Tip #2 - Keep meals simple and colorful. Sometimes we can overcomplicate things in our minds before we even take action. You don't need any weird ingredients or to follow complicated recipes to eat a healthy vegan diet. Whether you love to cook or prefer to find things already premade, ensure you have one main component that is filling, such as a starch (oats, whole wheat pasta or bread, rice, potatoes, polenta, etc.) and add as much color to it as you can in the form of fruits and veggies.

Tip #3 - Load up on healthy snacks. Since plant foods tend to be lower in calories than animal products, make sure that you fuel up often. It may take you some time to get used to this new way of eating, so to ensure you aren't ever stuck hungry without options around, keep something on hand at all times like a baggie of nuts and dried fruit, veggies with hummus, apples with nut butter, or a Larabar.

Meal Prep Tips

Many people are moving from one to-do list to the next, balancing work and family life, and often taking shortcuts when it comes to our health – especially when it comes to diet. Believe me, I can relate!

We have the best of intentions, but at the end of a long, hectic day, we find ourselves reaching for whatever is easy and quick, like junky fast food or store-bought frozen dinners. One of the best ways to avoid these pitfalls is to practice the art of preparing healthy ingredients, meals, and snacks in large batches for one or two time blocks during the week. While such a preparation might take some planning and an investment in time, the result will be time and money saved over the long run.

By prepping key ingredients and recipes ahead of time, those healthy foods will be ready for you during those busy weekdays. There's nothing better than reaching in the fridge and grabbing some already cut fruit, a mason jar of overnight oats, a pre-cooked veggie burger, or a homemade bowl of soup that can be reheated in the time it takes to load your favorite show on Hulu.

Buddha bowls and salads can be tossed together in minutes if the right ingredients are at hand. Lunches and dinners come together without having to put that much thought into it after a hectic day. It makes life so much easier! As an added bonus, your grocery bill will be lower since you're only stocking up on items you need for the meals you already planned. And as if you needed another reason to grab your free copy of the Endless Plant-Based Food Guide over at www.eatinglikeyougiveadamn.com/guide, it just so happens to have everything you need to get your new rebellious, albeit compassionate lifestyle kicked off easily and deliciously.

Here is some advice for helping you prepare healthy vegan foods for your busy week:

1. Plan ahead

Before you head to the grocery store, make a menu for the week, then check your pantry and refrigerator to review what ingredients you have on hand and what you are running low on. You may even want to keep a list of all the ingredients you stock in your kitchen as you toss out an old item with animal ingredients and replace it with a new vegan friendly item. There are a number of convenient apps for your phone or tablet that can help you manage your recipe lists.

2. Create a system that works for you

There are many creative ways to plan your meals on the fly. Here are some popular ones:

- Choose themes for each night – Monday may be Mexican Night, Tuesday Asian Night, Wednesday Italian Night, Thursday Burger Night, Friday Pizza Night, and so on.

- Cook meals that can be combined with new ingredients – Monday's chili can be used to top baked potatoes on Wednesday. Tuesday's tempeh "bacon" can be used as a pizza topping on Thursday and as a Buddha bowl ingredient for lunch on Friday. Quinoa can be served with veggies and beans one day, and added to your oatmeal or soup on another day. The possibilities are endless.

3. Shop weekly

Weekly shopping ensures that your produce stays fresh, and it minimizes waste. It is also much easier to plan meals for seven days than for an extended period of time.

Choose a day of the week to shop and schedule time for menu planning before then. For instance, you may do grocery shopping on Friday and place everything inside the fridge until Sunday when batch cooking and prepping is more convenient.

4. Batch cook and prep:

Buy a variety of fresh, seasonal fruit every week

- Strawberries, apples, pears, blueberries, raspberries, peaches, and grapes are best to wash right before you consume them. You don't want to wash fruit ahead of time or it may get moldy.

- Watermelons, cantaloupe, honeydew, pineapple, and mango are all great examples of fruits that can be cut up ahead of time and placed in sealed containers.

- Freeze some of your ripe bananas. These are key ingredients for smoothies, "nice cream," and more.

Create a "salad bar" in your fridge

- Slice veggies and store them in containers. Carrots, cucumbers, bell peppers, scallions, broccoli, cauliflower and celery are great toppings for your salad or Buddha bowls.

- Stock up on baby greens that are already pre-washed and ready to go, and wash and break up.

- Sauté mushrooms and onions and keep them in a container for tossing in hearty salads, Buddha bowls, wraps, on top of veggie burgers, etc.

Make a big pot of soup:

- Soup is an easy meal to prepare as everything goes in one pot. Switch it up and cook a different soup for each week.

Make a big pot of chili

- Chili is versatile and can be eaten in so many different ways: alone, over grains, on top of potatoes, over tortilla chips, etc.

Make a "Burger of the Week"

- Double or triple the recipe for your chosen burger of the week to make from scratch. Cook some to be eaten that week, and freeze others to be saved for a later time.

- Dress up your Beyond Burger with different themes each week, like American Classic, Mushroom and Daiya Swiss, and Western Barbeque. And, switch things up with a Filet-O-Fishless sandwich with homemade tartar sauce using an eggless mayo and Fishless Filets from Gardein.

Cook a large batch of grains

- Brown rice, quinoa, pasta, millet, buckwheat, and wild rice can be used to make soups, casseroles, bowls, and veggie burgers, or they can be enjoyed with beans and veggies.

Bake a bunch of potatoes

- Scrub some potatoes and sweet potatoes and put them in the oven at 400°F to bake for about 30-40 minutes or until you can stick a fork through them.

You can whip them out on a busy weeknight and serve them stuffed with steamed veggies, leftover chili, or as a side dish.

Marinate and cook up tempeh and tofu

- Slice tempeh into strips and tofu into steaks and marinate in a smoky "bacon" or Asian marinade for a few hours. Then fry them in a non-stick skillet and store them in the fridge for quick sandwiches, wraps and Buddha bowls.

Make some breakfast recipes

- If you make Sunday brunch, just double or triple the recipes to eat throughout the week. Popular recipes to batch cook for breakfast are pancakes, tofu scramble, overnight oats and granola.

Don't Like Cooking?

There are many meal delivery services that cater to vegans, and most of them include whole-foods, organic, and well-rounded meals. Some arrive to your home already chef prepared, like Veestro in the U.S., or All Plants in Great Britain. Another option is to have recipes with ingredients pre-measured delivered to your door, so there's little thought or planning ahead. Just follow the included recipes to whip up great meals. Purple Carrot is a great example in the U.S., and Fresh-n-Lean in Ontario, Canada.

6

Anticipate Your Obstacles

"Our greatest happiness does not depend on the condition of life in which chance has placed us, but is always the result of a good conscience, good health, occupation, and freedom in all just pursuits." Thomas Jefferson

No matter if you have just started making changes towards an exclusively plant-strong diet today or have been successful at it for a while, there are bound to be challenges that pop up every now and then. You will want to prepare ahead of time for the things you can control. Taking just a few minutes to take stock of what you have on hand, and imagining how you anticipate your day playing out will often save you from the attack of the hangry monster.

Time, money, dining out and social events are the top obstacles the new rebels for compassion run up against in the beginning stages of compassionate eating. No matter what obstacles you are presented with, revisiting your Big Why will help you stay the course until you find a resource, like a friend, book, blog post, podcast or film, that can outline the solution you might be looking for.

Cost

It's a common misconception that a plant-exclusive lifestyle jacks up the grocery bill. And no matter your household size, it really depends on two simple factors: where you shop and what you splurge on.

According to a 2015 poll by the Vegetarian Resource Group, the largest concentration of vegans is in the sub $50,000 income range. This might come as a surprise to some because it is assumed that veganism is reserved for the afflu-ent, but there are in fact more vegans in the lower end of the income range than the higher end. Parenthetically, the aver-age American earns $54,000.

Some of the most filling and fiber-packed plant foods that become the base ingredient for many of your meals are also some of the cheapest things in the store, like beans, rice, oats, potatoes, cabbage, and whole wheat pasta. Additionally, when you find yourself at restaurants where meat is usually the star of the show, the vegan options are always the cheap-est options on the menu. Even if you build yourself a meal full of vegetable side items a la carte.

If you're used to couponing, you won't find a lot of cou-pon savings for whole plant foods as you would for many processed nutrient-weak items in your local paper. Pay closer attention to the coupons and sales for food items. If they are a food source that is as close to being in its whole state as nature intended and full of fiber, then you're golden. Those are the health promoting foods you want more of and that's where you want to focus the bulk of your spending. If the item is processed from its whole form and packaged, and you can't easily identify the ingredients as those that you would actually consume individually, then ditch the coupon, as well as the food. Get addicted to real food, not savings parading as a food bargain today when it can make you fat and sick later.

While the government has played a key role in keeping the cost of poor quality meat, dairy and eggs affordable for consumers, don't forget the true cost of those items as it relates to your Big Why. You may have become used to a feeling of satisfaction from a fast food meal, Betty Crocker recipe, or Lean Cuisine costing you only a few bucks. But as you learn to examine the nutritional impact of those cheap, processed foods, you will find that they are not at all nutritious when compared to a simpler plant-based meal: like rice and beans with a big salad, a baked potato stuffed with lentils and steamed veggies, vegetables smothered in cashew cheese sauce, or a colorful stir fry. Shift your beliefs about what cheap food actually is and what it's costing you, and build your meals around the cheapest filling ingredients first. You can learn more about building delicious and nutritious plant-based bowls and plates on any budget by going to www.eatinglikeyougiveadamn.com/guide and downloading your free Endless Plant-Based Food Guide.

If you're used to spending $15 on a bag of frozen fish fillets or hunk of red meat for the week, transfer that amount in buying nuts, seeds and produce like dark leafy greens, broccoli, cabbage, apples, bananas, and even frozen fruits and vegetables. Find a local farmer's market or produce stand. Many times the produce comes off the same truck that is delivered to your local grocer, but the savings are worth the extra stop. Head to your local produce stand on their delivery days to initially stock up on fruits and vegetables before hitting the grocery store for the other meal ingredients on your list. You may find that when you're surrounded by only fruits and vegetables at affordable prices that you end up being inspired to buy more of those while crossing off some of the processed foods from your grocery list.

And finally, learn how to reduce your use of vegan transition foods like packaged cheeses, butter, mayo, ice cream and faux meats. They typically average $5-$8 each, whereas the cost of making these foods from a simple recipe is far lower, and in most cases, much healthier. Let these items become occasional treats, or splurges, while the majority of your meals are made using whole foods closest to their natural state.

Time

We all get the same amount of hours, minutes, and seconds in every day. And, we always find the time for the things we consider most important to us. If your plan was to begin your day at the gym, work a full day at the office (including a working lunch meeting), rush to your important dinner plan, tuck you kids into bed and read them a story, and finish a research paper before the deadline at midnight...and then your number one idol in the whole world called and said they needed to meet with you today, or something just as equally shocking comes up. What would you do? You would likely re-prioritize your whole day to include the new thing that just became highly important to you.

This is where your Big Why comes in. Your Big Why is the reason making time to plan your meals is a top priority. Whether you make the time each day of the week to plan and prep your meals, or just one block of time on one day of the week, etch it in stone on your schedule. And if your idol does call, make sure you meet up where good vegan food is served.

Instead of looking for "more time," try finding something you can do less of. For many Americans, that can mean spending less time either in front of the tv or at the workplace. Don't forget to grab your free copy of the Endless Plant-Based Food Guide at www.eatinglikeyougiveadamn.com/guide to save you even more time when planning out meals and grocery runs. In this guide, I have mapped out every possible plant-based option to build your meal and displayed it in such a way that you can spend less time thinking about what to eat and more time enjoying your food.

And, if you can buy yourself some time with money, try your local grocers online shopping and delivery service. Or, have pre-measured ingredients for several meals delivered to your door through a subscription from a plant-based meal delivery service like Purple Carrot or Veestro.

"I am not 100% vegan today but I know that one day I will be. When I was young I didn't really understand what it meant to be vegan so I certainly didn't imagine that I would aspire to be one. My first experience was just over 6 years ago...I decided to eat vegan for 30 days. I had more energy, was INSTANTLY able to run further with no trouble breathing and just felt overall amazing. I went to a family party on the last day and I had the traditional "party foods" including a piece of meat. Less than 30 minutes later I could feel the effects of that meal. Fast forward to a year ago, I was feeling pretty lousy and knew that my diet was one of the major reasons. I'm raising 3 small children, homeschooling them and running a business, so I subscribed to a vegan meal delivery service. I live in a very rural area, so vegan choices are RARE and I'm surrounded by dairy farms. My husband grew up on a dairy farm so all of these things make it challenging for me to just switch all at once. Becoming a vegan is a journey for me and I'm glad to be further ahead than I was a year ago. I know that even making the changes I already have that I'm making an impact."

Jessica Mierzwa - Forestville, NY

Dining Away from Home

Although finding more vegan options in mainstream restaurants is getting better because of the ever increasing demand, there are still many restaurants that are behind the times and offer only a few vegan options. If you eat out often, it can become tiring in eating the same single vegan meal over and over again, or to order fries and plain salad because they don't have any other noticeable vegan options on the menu. Then, there are some restaurants that can't even tell you if something is vegan or not because they don't know what "vegan" means. So what you should do?

Tip #1: Research and plan ahead
Use the Happy Cow app to find restaurants with vegan options nearby. If there are no vegan restaurants in your city, pick out an ethnic restaurant like Asian, Italian, Indian, or Mexican. Ethnic restaurants tend to have a lot more vegan variety than other restaurants.

For example:
Asian - veggie sushi rolls, miso soup, veggie fried rice (without egg), veggie spring rolls, tofu stir fry with rice or noodles.
Italian - pasta marinara, veggie pizza (without cheese), salad with oil and vinegar.
Indian- vegetable samosas and pakoras, chana masala or lentil dal with basmati rice.
Mexican - chips, guac and salsa, veggie fajitas, tacos, and burritos, rice and beans (ask if beans are made without animal lard).

Tip #2: Look up the restaurant's menu online
If your friends have picked the restaurant, find the menu online on their website, Facebook page or Yelp. If you can't

find the menu, make a quick call and see if they have any vegan options. If they don't know what "vegan" means, politely explain to them that you don't consume any animal products. If they don't offer anything vegan, ask if the chef could fix something for you. The chef is usually happy to do that because they like to make something out of the ordinary. Plus, you've created a new awareness for the chef to consider adding the vegan item to their menu.

Tip #3: Ask about substitutes
Most restaurants have vegetarian options, which can easily be made vegan. Ask if the dairy or egg can be removed from the dish or replaced with a vegan ingredient (for example, they can replace butter with oil). Many dressings in restaurants contain animal ingredients, so be sure to ask about a dressing you think might be vegan.

Tip #4: Get creative with side dishes
Most restaurants offer many different sides that are vegan, or can be prepared vegan if you ask for no butter, sour cream, cheese, etc. If you order sides like a baked potato, rice, beans, salsas and veggies, you can have a pretty balanced meal.

Tip #5: Eat before you go
If you know that the options will be very limited (for example, if you're going to a steakhouse or wing place), eat something nourishing beforehand and order a drink or a snack when you're at the restaurant.

When traveling on a plane, be sure to carry the snacks you like, for example nuts and fruit. This could also include either a sandwich or quinoa salad. On long flights with meals, most airlines will accommodate a vegan meal if you call ahead within a certain number of days before your departure. Be sure to check with your airline when you book your trip.

Many layovers happen in big city airports where vegan food is plentiful, or at least you can modify the vegetarian options. But it's always good to be prepared by looking up the restaurants at your layover location before you arrive so you aren't running around looking at the options when you're on a tight schedule.

Before your trip to other countries, Google search "guide to eating vegan in Munich/Dublin/Madrid/Bangkok" or wherever you are headed. You are likely to find blogs and articles from other generous vegans who have already charted the territory and provide great recommendations and tips, which is a huge time saver. And if you are unable to find this kind of helpful information for your intended destination, be sure to have access to a stove and fridge when you book your lodging. That way, you can shop for your plant-based groceries at the local markets and experiment with the local flavors.

Social Events

Whether it's a family gathering, a friend's birthday party, a concert or barbeque, the vegan options can be quite slim. To best prepare yourself and to show off what a savvy rebel you are, arrive with delicious plant-based food and be sure to take enough to share. This can be something you have made by yourself at home, or something you have picked up premade from a vegan friendly grocer like Whole Foods. If you're going to a grill out, simply bring your own favorite meatless patties or dogs, or make ahead some seasoned veggie and tofu skewers.

Not only will you be eating something you know you like, but you will be saving yourself from a desperate search for something substantial at the event. Trust me, this is coming from a gal who was caught eating a hotdog bun with just mustard and relish while onlookers criticized about how hard it must be to be vegan. It's actually not when we show up prepared with deliciousness that defy stereotypes, and in the end, other non-vegans want to steal. If you're needing ideas on what to take to your next event, be sure to download your free copy of the Endless Plant-Based Food Guide at www.eatinglikeyougiveadamn.com/guide for planning the perfect dish everyone can enjoy.

Another situation you may run into is turning down something that someone has offered you that isn't vegan. In the past, I have felt ashamed that I may have hurt my host's feelings by turning down their signature dish after becoming aware of them cooking all day, and putting their love into that meal for the enjoyment of others. Some cooks even have a sneaky way of making you feel guilty for not trying their food. If you find yourself in this situation, find something on the table that you can eat. Even if it's a plain side dish and some bread. And be sure to tell the host how wonderful it is and how grateful you are to have been invited to join everyone.

Keep in mind that there are many people in the world who can't or won't eat something for religious, allergy, or ethical reasons, and others have to be accepting of that. The host wouldn't have their feelings hurt if their Muslim guest declined the dish containing pork. In fact, as a good host, if they knew their Muslim friend would be sitting at the table they would feel more inclined to serve something more appropriate that everyone could enjoy. This is an example to keep in mind as a social rebel for compassion.

So, here are a few things you can do to avoid having these awkward encounters on the spot.

Tip #1: Let the host know ahead of time that you eat a plant exclusive diet. Most people will be happy to prepare something without animal ingredients for you.

Tip #2: Offer to contribute a vegan dish to share. If the host is unfamiliar with vegan food, say you'd like to help by making a delicious plant-based dish to add to the table. Find out the theme of the host's meal and prepare something that would go well with it.

Tip #3: In place of dessert, ask for coffee or tea without milk instead. Or pleasantly surprise the host by bringing a batch of your favorite vegan cookies to share.

If you're looking for tips on handling social pressures and answering questions about your plant-strong lifestyle without offending anyone during social events, that topic is covered in chapter 9.

7

Learn Basic Nutrition

*"Everything in food works together to create health or disease.
The more we think that a single chemical characterizes a
whole food, the more we stray into idiocy."*
Dr. T. Colin Campbell

I learned more about the basics of human nutrition during
my transition to eating plant-exclusive than I ever did over
my entire life as an everyday consumer of what I thought
were healthy animal products. The moment I decided to stop
eating foods that were derived from animals, I made the time
to figure out how to do it healthfully so that my livelihood
would never be compromised. I later figured out that if I didn't
come to the dinner table armed with statistical justifications
for my vegan choices, I would be subjecting myself to teasing
for being so soft about my reverence for animals. Sheesh.

I freaked at first about giving up certain animal based
"health foods" only because everywhere I looked there would

always be advertisements and articles sending me messages that foods like salmon, yogurt and eggs were necessary for my health. I needed to dig up an alternative argument on what I had been conditioned to believe so that I could look at the evidence critically and make my own informed choices about whether or not to allow some animal products for my own health. What I uncovered in that process were some compelling statistics advocating for a plant-based diet for optimal health while also realizing everything I thought I knew about eating animals, milk, and eggs for my health was dead wrong. I list resources in the back of this book that explain in more detail the positive impacts to one's health as a result of eating a plant-exclusive diet as well as the health implications of consuming popular animal products.

Despite the popular slogans fed to us by celebrities hired to make the meat, egg and dairy industries sexy, milk does not do a body good, eggs are not so incredible, and white meat is not actually healthier than any other form of dead animal flesh.

It's compelling to learn about some of the healthiest and longest lived people on the planet today living in various regions of the world called Blue Zones where the predominant source of nutrients location-wide come from dark leafy greens, legumes, whole grains, and colorful fruits and vegetables.

One thing I also find interesting is that the healthiest and longest lived people around the world don't obsess over counting calories or nutrients, or follow any of the popular diets that have any sort of marketable name. Which further illustrates that when we are eating mostly whole plant-based foods like our bodies were designed to function optimally on, we don't need to concern ourselves with nutrition labels, counting points or being strict about our macronutrients.

While nutrition information mixed with opinions and biases can be dizzying at times because, let's face it, that's what we are mostly subjected to, what we do need to pay attention to are a few key elements that everybody should know about our food, not just vegans.

The Macros

Protein

Have you noticed that the culinary world refers to all animal flesh as "protein?" I love to indulge in cooking shows from time to time, but I cringe when they refer to a single fleshy food as "the protein." It appears to me that this anesthetizing euphemism for an animal's body is an echo of an old way of seeing a balanced plate as an animal derived protein, a starch and bit of vegetable on the side. We should remember that culinary artists are not typically concerned with nutrition.

Almost all food, including food from the plant kingdom, contain protein. But you're likely not to hear that on television or read that in a popular cooking magazine. Which is just one reason why everyone is so profoundly confused today about this single, albeit important macronutrient.

So what do we need to know about protein as rebels for compassion, or as someone flirting with a plant-exclusive lifestyle?

While nutrition experts continue to battle the pervasive notion in our society that meat, dairy and eggs are synonymous with "protein" just because they contain higher concentrations of it, you and I need to be clear about the fact that protein deficiency is virtually nonexistent in industrialized countries. In fact, according to a 2013 study published in the Journal of the Academy of Nutrition and Dietetics, most American and European adults eat substantially more protein than the recommended amount — averaging more than 100 grams of protein per day when the average requirement is just 42 grams.

If you're eating a variety of whole plant foods, it's almost impossible to consume too little protein. The only people who are truly deficient in protein tend to have diets that are deficient in many important nutrients. For instance, those who aren't eating enough calories — which is a life-threatening concern for people who don't have enough food to eat. Additionally, alcoholics, addicts and people with eating disorders such as anorexia are known to fall prey to health complications by protein deficiency.

But in the industrialized world where starvation is relatively rare, inadequate protein consumption is almost unheard of. If you eat 2,400 calories in a day and 15% of your calories are coming from protein, you'll be eating 90 grams of protein.

Researchers are beginning to understand that far more people may be suffering from getting too much protein, than suffering from getting too little. A 2003 research review published in The American Journal of Clinical Nutrition confirmed that diets lower in meat consumption lead to greater longevity. The longer a person's adherence to a plant-strong diet, the lower their risk of mortality and the higher their life expectancy.

Rather than being hyper obsessed about getting enough protein, folks should be more concerned about fiber deficiency. The recommended amount of fiber is 25-30 grams per day and most Americans eat about 10-15 grams. And it's surprising for many to learn that our early ancestors were foragers who actually ate close to 100 grams of fiber per day, and not nearly the amount of dead animal flesh that is advertised by today's version of a paleo plate.

A whole foods vegan diet provides a healthy amount of soluble and insoluble fiber which is essential for reducing the risk of colon cancer, breast cancer, heart disease, diabetes, obesity, and stroke. It also helps control cholesterol and blood sugar levels, and it binds toxins, mercury and lead, which is mostly accumulated in animal fat.

And if getting complete protein as a vegan is of concern, rest easy because the position of the Academy of Nutrition and Dietetics is that protein from a variety of plant foods eaten during the course of a day supplies enough essential amino acids when caloric requirements are met.

Single sources of complete proteins - meaning they include an adequate proportion of all nine of the essential amino acids required for human health - include soybeans, tofu, tempeh, quinoa, buckwheat and Ezekiel 4:9 sprouted bread.

But even if you never include these foods in your daily repertoire, consuming a varied diet from all the food groups of the plant kingdom, you'll have your bases covered by way of foods that complement each other's amino acid profiles. And no, they don't need to be consumed at the same time as it was once thought. But, by some divine coincidence, many are preferred to be served together anyway.

Some examples of commonly combined foods that contain complete protein include toast with nut butter, hummus with pita bread or whole grain crackers, rice and beans (in a bowl, wrap, taco, etc.), and tofu or edamame stir fry served with rice or noodles.

So, if you are eating a well-rounded healthy diet full of a variety of nutrients and fiber, you do not need to be concerned about getting enough protein.

Carbs

Sometimes people avoid carbohydrates because they think they're fattening. This is a common misunderstanding thanks to, you guessed it, industry profiteers who bank on keeping you confused.

But once you begin to pay attention, you'll find there are carbs that in their whole and unprocessed form are good for you, but have been awarded a blanket labeling of "bad" and "fattening" simply because they can be turned into a fattening food high in calories and lacking in nutrition, like potatoes deep-fried in oil to make French fries and potato chips. If you were to take that potato, bake it, and stuff it with steamed broccoli, peppers and black beans, the fiber and nutrient packed potato is of no big fat concern.

Or, how about those relatively innocent carbs that are turned into vehicles for high calorie butter and cheese, like pizza, bread, and pasta?

It's actually the high-fat oils, butters, and cheeses that we pair with our processed carbs that really pack in the calories. In fact, gram for gram, fat contains more than twice the calories of carbohydrates. Weight gain will occur anytime we eat more calories than we burn. And joyfully, it's rather hard to overeat on a plant-based diet when the focus is put on whole foods that are naturally high in carbs and low in added fat. And, carbohydrates have less calories per gram than fat, therefore, they fill you up faster.

Here's where most of the confusion comes from...there is a difference between simple carbs and complex carbs in the way they are utilized by the body.

Simple carbohydrates, such as added sugars, syrups, and white flour break down fast, cause blood sugar rise, and in high consumption causes insulin resistance and weight gain. The exception here is fruit, which comes with health-boosting fiber, vitamins, minerals, and phytochemicals when consumed whole - and not as a container of juice.

In contrast, complex carbohydrates, like whole wheat, brown rice, vegetables and whole fruit come with a load of fiber which keeps you full longer, break down slowly, balance out your blood sugar and fuel your muscles with energy.

According to the Physicians Committee for Responsible Medicine, *fiber-rich carbohydrates* provide most of the calories in a *healthy* diet and are the main fuel for the brain and muscles. And about three-quarters of daily calories should come from complex carbohydrates for optimal health and weight.

The role that complex carbohydrates play in human health is too important to pass up. Many carbohydrate rich foods like sweet potatoes, beans, lentils, berries, bananas, oats, whole wheat, barley, rye and quinoa promote good health by delivering vitamins, minerals, fiber, and a host of important phytonutrients while providing the body with glucose, which is converted to energy used to support bodily functions and physical activity.

"Fad diets often lead people to fear carbohydrates. But the research continues to show that healthy carbohydrates–from fruits, vegetables, beans, and whole grains–are the healthiest fuel for our bodies," said director of clinical research for PCRM Hana Kahleova, M.D., Ph.D.

Fat

I remember when I was a teen and had begun to pay attention to my figure. I was addicted to sweets. It was the sweets containing fat that became the devil to my waistline, or so I thought. So when my mom came home from the store with fat free Snack Wells cookies, Fig Newtons and low-fat ice cream, I couldn't get enough! This is an example of how as people we can often take things that bring us pleasure to extremes. As I've heard physician and expert on the effects of nutrition on disease Dr. John McDougall state: "People love to hear 'good news' about their bad habits."

Today, most of us who are interested even in the slightest on nutrition know that refined sugar was the "fattening" agent of the low-fat and fat free craze of the 90's. If you didn't yet know, sorry to burst your bubble (sorry, not sorry). More sugar was often added to replace the fat that was removed from processed foods in order for them to taste good and keep us coming back for more. But the bottom line is that it's still junk food, and marketers are going to find ways to make that junk food sound appealing enough for you to continue buying it.

We get that there are good fats and bad fats. The question is, what are healthy fat sources and where do we find them?

Animal-based fats, which contain a lot of saturated fat and cholesterol, are not only unnecessary for human health, they promote high LDL cholesterol, clogged arteries, inflammation, diabetes and heart disease. The human body can produce enough cholesterol on its own without needing dietary cholesterol from other sources. Fish, though promoted as a healthy source of omega fatty acids, is in fact one of the foods highest in cholesterol, as well as eggs and butter which also contain animal-based saturated fats.

Plant-based fats have no cholesterol. The plant-based kingdom is full of healthy fats, leaving little need for much else. While animal-based fats are associated with a higher risk of dying from heart disease and other causes according to research, plant-based monounsaturated fats — like those found in avocados, raw nuts and seeds, coconuts, olives and cacao are associated with a lower risk of dying. And in fact, healthy plant-based fats which are dense in nutrients are important for nervous system function, heart health, brain health, metabolism and digestion.

Oils are concentrated sources of calories and will often promote weight gain. Oils aren't necessary for health if you eat whole food sources of fats. However, oils such as hemp, olive and coconut do have more health benefits than other vegetable oils like corn and soy, which often contain GMO's, promote inflammation and may cause poor artery and heart health. It can feel funky at first to sauté your veggies in water or veggie broth instead of oil if you intend to avoid or simply cut back on it, but the outcome for your food is that it's still the same cooked result you were looking for while being kinder to your waistline.

The Micros

When animal-based foods are replaced with wholesome plant foods, something magical happens. We inevitably consume more micronutrients (vitamins and minerals), phytochemicals, antioxidants and anti-inflammatories than we ever did as constant meat, dairy, and egg eaters.

In my online vegan nutrition certification course for health coaches, I teach about the various colors of fruits and vegetables and their correlating micronutrients as well as the health benefits those nutrients provide. For example, bioactive phytochemicals in berries work to repair damage from oxidative stress and inflammation, while green fruits and vegetables are rich in lutein, isothiocyanates, isoflavones, and vitamin K — as well as folate, which is a nutrient especially important for pregnant women to consume to help prevent congenital disabilities.

But the two most common micronutrients that most people think vegan diets are lacking are calcium and iron.

We were taught since childhood that the best source of calcium for strong bones is milk. Bones need a complex set of ingredients to be healthy, not just calcium. Vitamin K and magnesium work hard to aid in calcium absorption and stabilization in the bone, making dark leafy greens a far better choice. Dairy is not only lacking in these nutrients, but according to a study in the British Medical Journal, cow's milk is known to leach nutrients from the bone.

The Physicians Committee for Responsible Medicine shows this is the latest in a plethora of studies showing not only that milk fails to protect bone health, but that plant-based nutrition is more effective for disease prevention.

Calcium is absorbed and utilized efficiently and effectively by our bodies from plant-based foods like greens, seeds, some nuts, and vegetables.

As for iron, if you eat legumes, nuts, seeds and green leafy veggies like kale on the regular, then you will be getting in your necessary iron.

A free tool I think is pretty badass to utilize is cronometer.com to log the food you eat. And not only will you see your macronutrient intake, but your mineral and vitamin intake as well. A balanced plant-based diet gives you more minerals and vitamins than the recommended daily value. And, with the cronometer tool you can determine if you indeed lack any necessary nutrition so you can be empowered to adjust your diet accordingly.

If you are still worried, speak with a doctor to get your vitamin and mineral levels checked.

Supplements

It's easy to see how removing meat, eggs and dairy from the diet is very rewarding to one's health. But what tends to happen with many people who "go vegan" is they rely on processed junk foods, and can sometimes ignore the need to supplement intelligently. This is not a limitation of the vegan diet, but represents the state of the world with depleted soil, indoor lifestyles and the need for convenience resulting in low vitamin intake.

Supplement only where necessary to prevent damaging your health and your wallet. The following list is what doctors and dietitians of plant-based nutrition recommend adding into not just a plant-based diet, but even non-vegan diets, too.

B12

Vitamin B12 is the only nutrient required for those eating plant-exclusive, but not for the reason most people think. It is a common misconception that this necessary vitamin comes from animals. Certain bacteria in the guts of animals make B12 from the soil and feces they ingest, so this necessary nutrient actually comes from the soil and not the animal. Historically, by eating "dirty" vegetables from the earth or foraging foods from the wild, humans ingested B12. But now, with modern farming and washing practices, dirt is no longer a viable source of B12 for most people.

B12 prevents nerve damage, protects the heart, and supports your overall energy level and immune system. B12 deficiency can be a danger to people who eat meat, too. Studies estimate that between 20-40% of people in developed countries have a B12 deficiency.

Instead of relying simply on fortified foods, like many non-dairy milks and nutritional yeast, it's wise to take a supplement that becomes your reliable source for this crucial nutrient. The official RDI in the United States is 4 micrograms per day. But Dr. Joel Fuhrman, a family physician and internationally recognized expert on nutrition and natural healing, and many other leading medical experts recommend taking 2,500 mcg of cyanocobalamin B12 once a week or at least 250 mcg daily to meet this essential need. Methylcobalamin is sometimes recommended by health professionals at a higher dose because some studies suggest that the body may absorb cyanocobalamin better than methylcobalamin, while other studies have found that the differences in absorption and retention are minimal. Additionally, if you're over 65, increase your dosage of vitamin B12 to 1,000 mcg daily as absorption decreases when we get older.

D3

It's estimated that 40-60% of the world's adult population doesn't get enough of the sunshine vitamin, making this the most common vitamin deficiency in the world today. Why? Because in the modern world, we spend most of our time clothed and indoors while our ancestors worked outdoors and didn't wear much clothing. Additionally, many of us live in northern climates with low sunshine levels, particularly in the winter months.

Vitamin D (which is technically a hormone) is famous for helping your body absorb calcium and other minerals, is crucial for the healthy functioning of your muscles, heart, brain, pancreas, and thyroid, protects you from getting the cold and flu, and reduces your risk of dementia and many kinds of autoimmune diseases.

For most who don't get a daily dose of about 30 minutes of sun exposure over the majority of their skin, a daily dose of 2,000 IU of vitamin D3 will ensure you get the right amount, according to the Vitamin D Council. Look for a vegan source from lichen as opposed to fish or lanolin from sheep's wool.

Omega Fatty Acids

The three primary omega-3 fatty acids are: ALA (alpha-linolenic acid), EPA (eicosapentaenoic acid) and DHA (docosahexaenoic acid). Although they are not considered essential in the diet, all three are critical to brain health, combating depression, stabilizing the rhythm of the heart, lowering triglycerides, helping prevent the most common types of cancer, and more.

The commonly recognized source for omega fatty acids are fish, but fish don't make these omegas. They get them from the plankton and algae that they eat. And many fish and fish oils also carry harmful toxins, like mercury, and are often rancid.

On an exclusively plant-based diet, you cut out the middle man (or, middle fish) by taking an algae-based supplement, which doesn't contain the bioaccumulation or biomagnification of dangerous toxins.

Vegan EPA and DHA are found mainly in sea vegetables and certain algae. Sea vegetables such as nori, wakame, kelp, agar and dulse are also rich in iodine, protein and antioxidants while being more sustainable than current fishing practices. These and other sea vegetables can be found in your local health food store, Asian market, or an online retailer like Amazon. But if you are not a fan of eating seaweed, which is commonly enjoyed in Japanese cuisine, you can obtain these vital nutrients in supplement form.

The human body can convert ALA from easily accessible plant foods to EPA and DHA, though the efficiency of conversion varies from person to person. Plant foods highest in ALA are ground flax seeds, ground chia seeds, canola oil, camelina oil, walnuts, and hemp seeds.

However, considering how important EPA and DHA are to human health, supplementation is probably a good idea for most people, vegan or not. How much do you need? There's no official recommendation, but experts suggest 250-500 milligrams combined EPA and DHA each day for healthy adults.

"Towards the end of 2015, I always felt sick and had this mysterious pain in an unfavorable and embarrassing place. Debilitating pain. They thought it was unrelated. I was going to have to live with this pain forever, so they said. My parents passed away from cancers before I was 40. I already had a scare at 24 with precancer in my breast, but nothing scared me like what I was about to go through.

Jan 28, 2016, I had my tubes tied. Dr wasn't expecting to find anything unusual since all was good just a few months prior. But they found suspicious precancerous cells.

March 17, 2016, I had a LEEP, a procedure to remove enough or all tissue to biopsy. In just 5 weeks, what was suspicious grew to be stage 3, a step below cancer. They said it was the most aggressive they've ever seen. They also found a very large fibroid tumor, that is in the way to see what is behind it. They need to remove it along with infected areas. 2nd opinion agreed.

I gave up meat and dairy at that moment. Literally over-night, or quicker.

May 10, 2016, at the age of 41, I had a full hysterectomy. I had a list of oncologists to contact before I was to leave the hospital, they were convinced I would have cancer. My tumor was so large, my doctor asked if he could bring in a different surgeon that he felt is better than him. I agreed. When I woke up, my doctor was surprised and told me that not only did the cells not spread, they didn't grow. I somehow stopped it. He asked what I did, and I told him I quit meat and dairy. He said don't ever go back.

P.S. the pain is gone...

More than a year later, with the support of a few good friends and fiance, and the help of an Instant Pot and Vita-mix, I'm an advocate of plant food being medicine. I may not stop from getting cancer, but I'm not going to feed it. It'll have to fight to thrive."

Staci Chabowski - Reno, NV

What to Eat (Ideally)

Modern nutritional science has proven that a diet dominated by unrefined plant food, even exclusively containing plant food, is superior for prevention and reversal of chronic disease. Eating plant-exclusive is not unusual, as we likely evolved from predominantly plant-eating ancestors millions of years ago and remain close genetic relatives to predominantly plant-eating primates. I believe, based on certain evidence from anthropologists, that in the environment of food scarcity we evolved in, humans adapted to do quite well with a wide range of foods. That being said, are we designed to eat some some meat, dirt or insects? Perhaps, but we don't need to in today's environment of overabundance and variety now that we are aware of the undesirable implications related to the consumption of animal protein.

Dr. Greger's latest book How Not To Die offers an easy suggestion for a healthy, balanced plant-exclusive lifestyle. He calls it the Daily Dozen, and he offers the recommended number of servings for each suggestion. This is based on his decades of analyzing evidence from hundreds of studies on nutrition, and he breaks down in easy to understand terms many of those studies at NutritionFacts.org for us who are not of the medical profession. Here's what the daily dozen looks like:

1. 3 servings of **Beans** - baked beans, soybeans, chickpeas, peas, kidney beans, tofu, hummus, etc.

2. 1 serving of **Berries** - raisins, grapes, blackberries, blueberries, cherries, raspberries, strawberries, etc.

3. 3 servings **Other Fruits** - apples, avocados, bananas, tomatoes, oranges, grapefruit, melons, lemons, limes, etc.

4. 1 serving of **Cruciferous Vegetables** - broccoli, cauliflower, kale, rocket/arugula, brussel sprouts, etc.

5. 2 servings of **Greens** - spring mix, kale, young salad greens, rocket/arugula, spinach, swiss chard, etc.

6. 2 servings of **Other Vegetables** - sweet corn, zucchini/courgettes, carrots, garlic, mushrooms, onions, pumpkin, sweet potatoes, etc.

7. 1 Tbsp. of **Flaxseeds**

8. 1 serving of **Nuts and Seeds** - peanut, almond, brazil, walnut, sunflower seeds, pumpkin seeds, chia seeds, etc.

9. 1 quarter teaspoon of Turmeric, plus any other **Spices** you love

10. 3 servings of **Whole Grains** - brown rice, wild rice, quinoa, oats, whole wheat pasta, etc.

11. 5 servings of **Drinks** - water, coffee, green tea, white tea, black tea, hibiscus tea, etc.

12. Ideally 90 minutes of **Exercise** daily of moderate activity, such as walking

Another idea that Dr. Greger shares is a simple way to determine what is healthy if there is ever any question. If someone were to ask if vegan pizza is considered healthy, Dr. Greger would simply ask "healthy compared to what?" If you are comparing a homemade pizza made from whole grain flour, vegetables and marinara sauce to a meat lover's pizza from Pizza Hut, then the answer is self evident if you are aware of the potential health implications of eating copious amounts of processed meat and cheese.

And how about burgers? Is a vegan Beyond Meat burger even healthy? If you are comparing raw apples to apple pie, meatless burgers to beef burgers, and nut cheeses to dairy cheeses, then the vegan version is the healthier choice when compared to its animal equivalent, based on the scientific evidence regarding the negative impacts of animal protein (visit nutritionfacts.org for a comprehensive list of studies).

Now, if you ask if a fully loaded meatless burger is healthier than a colorful, well balanced whole foods kale salad... then just smack yourself.

If creating a daily menu of a well-balanced plant strong meal is not yet your strong suit, head over to www.eatinglikeyougiveadamn.com/guide to grab your free copy of the Endless Plant-Based Food Guide which includes tons of wholesome omnivore approved vegan food and flavor combinations, as well as what a well-balanced plant-based meal looks like on your plate or in your bowl.

8

Enrich Your Environment

"Do the best you can until you know better. Then when you know better, do better." –Maya Angelou

On our mental and emotional journey to becoming more compassionate in our food choices, we can find ourselves at times surrounded by negativity. Ok, probably a lot of times. From meat, dairy and egg advertisements everywhere, to the folks you share your table with eating something you now see as a product of cruelty, and to the hostile debates on social media between opposing viewpoints about eating animals. And no matter if you are a newly budding rebel for compassion or have been a compassionate consumer for years, seeing images of animal cruelty pop up unexpectedly on your social media newsfeed can feel emotionally draining and, consequently, derail your whole day.

On top of that, it might feel a bit lonely in the beginning, especially if you don't know where to find other like-minded people in your community.

The good news is that there are so many wonderful changes taking place throughout the world every single day, and this in effect is progressing our human culture forward to a more compassionate and sustainable future. When we know where to look for this life affirming information, we will find many of the incredible signs in the global demand for plant-based vegan food, such as:

- Large food corporations, such as Tyson, are investing billions of dollars into innovative vegan food technology in support of a more sustainable food system. Tyson is an investor in Beyond Meat, Israeli clean meat startup Future Meat Technologies Ltd. and San Francisco-based cultured meat brand Memphis Meats. Tyson Foods CEO Tom Hayes said "If we can grow the meat without the animal, why wouldn't we?"

- Nestlé, the largest food company in the world, predicts that plant-based foods will continue to grow and this trend is "here to stay." And Dairy giant Danone invested $60 million in dairy-free products.

- According to a report by research firm GlobalData, only 1% of U.S. consumers identified as vegan in 2014. And in 2017, that number rose to 6%. That's a 600% increase in just 3 years!

- According to the world's leading marketing intel agency Mintel, Germany accounted for 15% of global vegan product introductions between July 2017 and June 2018, followed by the UK at 14% and the US at 12%, making Germany the leading face in the vegan movement.

- The preliminary draft of Canada's new Food Guide, released in 2017 by the Canadian government, favors plant-based foods, making it possible for other government food guides to avoid influence from animal-food industry groups and to promote a scientifically grounded whole foods, plant-based dietary pattern.

- In Great Britain, the number of vegans quadrupled between 2014 and 2018, according to research organized by the Food Standards Agency. And 56% of Brits surveyed in 2017 report they adopted vegan buying behaviors such as buying vegan products and checking if their toiletries are cruelty-free.

- Italy had the fastest growing vegetarian population over 2011-2016 with a growth of 94.4%, According to Euromonitor International.

- Australia is the third-fastest growing vegan market in the world with the number of food products launched carrying a vegan claim rose by 92% between 2014 and 2016.

- New dietary guidelines released by the Chinese government encourage the nation's 1.3 billion people to reduce their meat consumption by 50%. In Hong Kong, 22% of the population reports practicing some form of a plant-based diet. Research predicts that China's vegan market will grow more than 17% between 2015 and 2020.

- With 400 vegan and vegan-friendly kitchens catering to most of Israel's high percentage of vegans, Tel Aviv is dubbed as "vegan capital of the world." Since 2012, the explosion of plant-based restaurants has transformed Israel's population of just eight million into the largest vegan nation, per capita, in the world.

- The line of 20 Wicked Kitchen vegan meals was rolled out at 600 UK Tesco stores at the start of 2018 and sold more than 2.5 million units in the first 20-week period ending in May 2018 — more than double the company's sales projections. "Selling more than double predictions is huge for a new brand, vegan or not," said Wicked food innovator Derek Sarno.

- With the fast rise in demand for plant-based milks, Elmhurst Dairy, a century-old US company whose dairy milk could be found everywhere from Manhattan Starbucks cafés to 1,400 different public schools city-wide, reinvented itself as a plant milk start-up in 2016 because – in its CEO's words – "milk has sort of gone out of style."

- Egg company Cal-Maine Foods reported a $74 million dollar loss due to vegan alternatives in 2017.

- An Oxford University study in June 2018 - which is the most comprehensive analysis to date of the damage farming does to the planet - found that 'avoiding meat and dairy is the single biggest way to reduce your impact on Earth' as animal farming provides just 18% of calories but takes up 83% of our farmland.

With statistics like these, it's hard to argue that we are alone on this self-propelled journey to becoming a compassionate and conscious consumer. But, I get it. It can still feel a bit lonely sometimes when the majority of the people you spend the most time with haven't yet figured out what's going on in the world of food like you have.

The key to keeping your sanity when your co-worker keeps laying non-vegan donuts under your nose, your friends keep wanting to meet up for dinner at a wing place, and your annoying cousin shouts "bacon!" every time you visit your family, is to surround yourself in positive messages that affirm your compassionate values while massaging a more positive mindset. And with a more positive mindset, you will ooze those good vibes onto others in your daily interactions - making omnivores everywhere wonder what on earth you're eating, drinking or smoking to be so joyful all the time (and where can they get some for themselves). Here are some ways to do that:

Get Savvy Online

Our faces are mostly plastered to our computer screens, phones and tablets. So it can be a huge benefit to make adjustments to what you do see and don't see in your social media platforms. Fortunately, this is easy to adjust.

In your journey to learning more about the hard truths of our food system, you may have opted into groups on Facebook, subscribed to YouTube channels, and began following people and organizations on Instagram and Twitter. If you end up with mostly positive, informative and uplifting content, great job! You probably don't need to change anything.

But, if you are seeing images, scare tactics and stories that make you feel anxious, depressed or ready to throw your iPhone into oncoming traffic, then you should consider making some adjustments.

If you have a friend on Facebook who tends to have a negative attitude towards veganism, or maybe they're the vegan stuck in the angry and evangelical stages of their journey and post images of animal cruelty while shaming their friends, you don't have to unfriend them altogether (unless you want to, of course). Simply unfollow them, and they'll never have to know.

Same with Twitter, Instagram and YouTube. If you find that you are following people who no longer add value to your day, simply unfollow them. Then, replace them with someone who does add value - like with inspirational quotes, useful communication tips, helpful cooking and shopping hacks, and uplifting images and stories about animals, the environment and improvements to health. This is what Eating Like You Give a Damn puts out into the popular social media channels, btw. Surprise, surprise.

Another thing to consider is tapping into the numerous daily positive changes in the world as they are happening. Consider setting up a Google Alert for "plant-based" and "vegan" to monitor the web for interesting new content. It will send you relevant world news to your inbox daily, weekly or monthly, depending on your preferences.

Online news channels like Plant Based News, Veg News, and Live Kindly are awesome outlets for seeing how the rising demand for vegan products is positively impacting the world. Opt-in to their mailing lists and follow them on social media to keep up with the many great advances in all things compassionate and sustainable.

Finally, find plant-based and vegan related podcasts to listen to and learn from. Podcasts are a great medium for up to the minute relevant content that you find useful and entertaining to you. Plus, you can get a sense of being in a community of like-minds with the host, guests and other listeners. This was a huge help to me when I lived overseas and felt disconnected from not just my American culture, but from my new vegan culture as well. I found new podcasts by searching on terms, like "vegan" and "plant-based," and listened to an episode of each one until I found my favorites.

Get Surprises in The Mail

Nothing makes me giddier these days after receiving something other than bills and junk mail in my mailbox. And when it's an occurring subscription, it gives me something to look forward to.

Since we spend so much time in front of the computer and phone screens, it can be a nice break on the eyes to thumb through beautiful and insightful magazines instead. And when it comes to the plethora of vegan and plant-based magazines that are available these days and which cover a wide range of interests from cooking to travel to fashion, you might just get inspired to do something you wouldn't have thought to search for online. For instance, I never imagined myself making vegan cheese from scratch, but the deliciously colorful display on Vegan Food and Living magazine and the easy instructions that only require 15 mins of prep time hooked me.

Plus, so many brands of vegan fashion, body care and unique travel destinations are on my radar that I likely wouldn't have found outside of my magazine subscriptions. I even found out about a vegan version of Airbnb called VegVisits with vegan hosts all over the world from a magazine. And when I do travel, these lightweight and thin publications make great travel companions. And, I love to "recycle" them when I'm done by gifting them to curious people I meet who may want a glimpse into compassionate living.

Another surprise that's fun to receive in your mailbox, and on your doorstep, are vegan subscription boxes. There are many different kinds depending on what you're into, such as snacks and treats like Urthbox, cruelty-free beauty products like Petit Vour, personal care and home cleaning essentials like Honest Company, and even entire healthy ready-made vegan meals delivered regularly to your door like Veestro. There's even Vegan Jerky of the Month Club and Vegan Wines wine club subscriptions that will ship these goodies right to your door! When it comes to discovering new vegan goodness, there's something for everyone ready to delight you in your mailbox or on your doorstep.

Get Social with Like-Minds

It's no surprise that because of the brave work of whistle-blowers who act today in the realms of animal agriculture, the environment, and health that the vegan movement is growing rapidly. But maybe you live in an area where you feel like you are the one and only rebel for compassion in your community. Good news, lovie. You're not. You just haven't found your local tribe yet.

Today's technology is a beautiful thing in many respects, however it has fostered people losing face-to-face connections outside of work. And it's time to put that technology to good use for connecting face-to-face in your area.

The need for human connection and shared values within close-knit social groups is primal, and it brings us all kinds of warm fuzzies and a sense of security when we are connected with people who share our beliefs, dreams, values and culture. If you feel like you are going it alone, it's time to utilize Facebook to get more like-minded people in your face. Here are some simple tips for finding and connecting with other rebels in your area.

There are meetup groups for just about everything around your zip code, and the Meetup app for your phone helps you search events that others with your shared interests are hosting. It could be anything like a wellness seminar, yoga retreat, vegan booze and bbq, plant-based running club or vegan dinner and discussion group. Many are held in health food stores, restaurants and at festivals. There are even fun annual and semi-annual vegfests and wellness expos to keep an eye out for.

Whatever event tickles your pickle, secure your spot and show up!

If you're the socially anxious type, beware that your brain may try to take you out of this by over analyzing things. "What if they don't like me? What if I don't like them? What if they're too militant or weird? What if...?" The reality is that all of your concerns may turn out to be true or completely untrue. But you'll never know who you could have met if you don't show up.

Facebook events are another popular way to discover unique meetups and events in your city. What's cool about showing your interest in these events, by simply clicking the Interested button, is that the algorithm will not only put more events and groups like it in your newsfeed to find easily from here on out, but you will also be surprised to see local people you are already connected with who are interested in the same event or group. This gives you a unique opportunity to reach out and make a plan to show up together and find more like-minded connections that way.

"I started my journey to becoming vegan about 22 years ago. I was in college and had become physically exhausted from lack of sleep due to my intense work/school schedule. My taste buds changed over the course of 6 months. I stopped eating steak, then ground beef, then chicken, and finally turkey. The last meat dish I ate was a turkey sandwich. I vowed not to eat meat anymore after eating that sandwich because it had a horrible taste. I was a lacto-ovo vegetarian for a year then I became a pescatarian. Over the years I have become very compassionate towards animals which solidified my desire not to eat meat. I have never been a fan of the taste of eggs so I rarely would eat them, but I loved eating cheese and gelato. A few months ago I watched 'What the Health"- that documentary helped me to realize that dairy cows suffer great abuse at the farms and throughout the process. I have been transitioning over to being vegan ever since then. Since doing so I have met many other people who are vegan and to my surprise I have quite a few friends whom are adopting a vegan diet as well which makes it very easy to socialize and dine out. I am so lucky to live in an area that has a plethora of very good vegan restaurants. I feel so much lighter and more satiated when I eat vegan. There are also health benefits to going vegan. I noticed a correlation between when I ate dairy and when I didn't prior to my menstrual cycle. When I ate dairy I would get cramps. The more dairy I would eat leading up my cycle the stronger the cramps would be. I used to get nausea as well during my cycle, however since eating vegan the nausea and cramps have ceased. I am loving the veggie life!"

Melissa Peavey - St. Petersburg, FL

If you feel plant-based events are too slim in your area, host one!

After becoming involved with other networking groups that were specific to my other interests, like personal and professional development, I built lasting relationships with people who weren't initially turned on by plant-based eating. But through getting to know me, they became accepting of my vegan lifestyle and open to seeing how my husband and I like to eat.

One day, my husband Dave and I decided to host a 'Veggin' Out with the Harters' event in our home and invited all the new friends we had made over that past year. We provided beer and wine and an awesome spread of vegan finger foods and snacks. We also showed off our Tower Garden full of lettuces, kale and herbs in our backyard and showed how we eat fresh off the Tower regularly.

We had about 13 friends and associates raving over vegan food, like "meatball" sliders, buffalo chik'n strips, bbq jackfruit sliders, and crabless stuffed mushrooms. We had a strict no-salad-or-hummus rule for this gathering! We wanted to show off to our friends who were meat eaters that eating compassionately doesn't have to mean giving up on the familiar taste and texture of comfort foods. They were very pleasantly surprised! And, after the delicious smorgasbord, they were all open to watching a video on YouTube with us called "101 Reasons to Go Vegan," which answered a lot of their questions about why Dave and I gave up eating animals - and much better than we could have answered them ourselves.

While we never expected anyone to change their point of view and adopt a compassionate lifestyle for themselves, it was very cool to see that we did in fact inspire some of those friends to learn more on their own to begin shifting to a mostly plant-based lifestyle for themselves. And to this day when we have gatherings with those members of our community who shared our Veggin' Out with us, we enjoy discussing many other shared interests without the usual vegan inquisition we get with other non-vegan groups. While we always love to share about our rebellious lifestyle with inquisitors, it is also pretty darn nice to not only be in communion with others who share the vision, but to know that we are kindly accepted by even those who don't.

Get Connected with Rescues

Have you ever talked to a rooster, and you'd swear he talked right back to you? Have you ever given a pig belly rubs, kissed a cow, or felt a hen purring as you pet her in your lap?

I couldn't say that I ever had until I discovered farm animal rescues and sanctuaries. Sure, I had been to petting farms as a kid, but never have I felt so spiritually connected to animals raised for food than when I visited a sanctuary and heard the stories of each individual animal while having the opportunity to interact and play them.

As a suburban and urban dweller with Southern roots, I hadn't noticed how accustomed to the concrete jungle I had become. Growing up with dogs, cats, hamsters, ferrets, guinea pigs and fish, I always had been aware, on some level, that each animal is an individual like us, and that they have their own personalities and quirks just as we do. I didn't grow up on a farm, and was never formally told to look upon any one animal as a pet, and the other as a meal. But even if I had, and based on other people's accounts who did grow up on farms and had an awakening later in life, I imagine I would still have the same blissful reaction today.

I never really saw farmed animals, unless they were grazing in a field as I drove down a highway or pecking in a neighbor's yard. So when I experienced meeting some of those farmed individuals after learning the horrific and destructive truths of animal agribusiness, I felt an overwhelming sense of joy for being their advocate and seeing them as individuals through the lens of compassion.

As a safe haven for rescued animals, sanctuaries are excellent replacements to traditional (yet unethical) family outings such as the zoo, aquariums, and petting zoos. If you have kids, nieces or nephews who love animals, chances are they are under the impression that the previously named animal "attractions" are a positive way to be present with animals. But today the public is seeing evidence of the cruelty and oppression towards the animals in captivity and on display. Even circuses have been banned from including exotic animals in their performances in many countries.

At an animal sanctuary, children and adults connect with four-legged and winged friends in a safe, non-invasive setting. Many rescued animals have heartbreaking backgrounds and near death experiences, reminding us that there is much work to be done to help shift our cultures mindset about eating them and using them for personal gain. Once they are taken to a rescue farm, they grow to enjoy the affection from their new animal friends and human visitors, and they love to cuddle, play and experience true freedom. The animals and their stories are the key to changing hearts, minds, and diets.

From your experience at a farm animal sanctuary you will consequently become a humane educator to your own friends and community as you share your personal experiences interacting with animals and the thoughts you develop on the relevant topics that interest you, such as animal agriculture; animal behavior, intelligence and emotional lives; wildlife conservation; or government policy and legislation for a more benevolent society. If you are a social learner like me, an animal sanctuary will be the perfect environment for your personal and spiritual growth.

Just by swapping the time and money you would have spent on a trip to the movies, going to a carnival or other fun outing with friends or family, visiting a rescue farm and supporting the social cause for compassionate living is one of the most fundamentally rewarding actions anyone can take.

I really can't describe the beautiful emotion that is felt when you enter a field and chickens come over to greet you, or when a goat follows you around because he wants to hang out and be buds, or when a gentle cow meets your eye and swearing to yourself that he or she is smiling while accepting an apple from your hand. It really is nourishing for the soul.

With all of the craziness and disconnectedness in the world today, there is something truly magical about spending time with animals who want nothing taxing from you, accept for maybe a treat and a few belly rubs.

9

Communicate with Confidence

"I am in favor of animal rights as well as human rights. That is the way of a whole human being." Abraham Lincoln

Hope meets up with a mix of friends and new acquaintances for dinner and drinks. After placing her order and making sure the server knows that she wants her meal to be vegan, someone from the table inquires about the length of time she has been vegan, and questions how could she ever give up cheese or bacon. Because Hope is several months into her vegan journey, she feels equipped to provide a polite yet informative answer. So she begins by sharing a few facts about the impact of eating meat, dairy and eggs on animals, the environment, and human health. Hope stated the kind of facts that she was sure the non-vegan acquaintance, Kris, would respond to, just as she did when she first learned about them, like any rational, caring person would.

For reasons unclear, however, the words didn't land quite right, since Kris engaged in defending the status quo of eating animals. Indeed, Kris counteracted every fact that Hope had raised: Their grandfather ate meat and cheese every day and lived to be 92. Their neighbor raises happy chickens in their backyard, and since chickens lay eggs anyway, what's wrong with eating them? And, they had a friend who was vegan and got sick, so he isn't vegan anymore.

Hope felt frustrated and bewildered by the irrationality behind Kris's justifications. Keeping in mind how important it is for more people to experience an awakening about eating animals as she did, Hope then made an attempt to rephrase her thoughts and included more facts to support her way of thinking to be understood more clearly. But her words seemed to fall on deaf ears, and sadly they were perceived solely as her own personal opinion.

Heated and emotional, Hope wanted to find Kris's capacity for displaying empathy, and so she began by describing graphic abuses towards animals in agribusiness, together with the catastrophic effects on human health and the planet. But Kris chalked all this up to Hope being melodramatic and embellishing the truth in order to push her vegan agenda. Both Hope and Kris were at a bitter stalemate.

Tune in to Turn 'Em On

I've seen this kind of story play out time and time again, and I've seen how utterly defeated it can make someone feel who is living a vegan lifestyle. And while we sometimes may feel like beating hypnotized people over the head with facts in hopes that they'll get the message and show some reverence for the violence and destruction we witness in the name of cheeseburgers, bacon and hot wings, we want to equally be successful in our level headed communication of opposing the status quo.

Sometimes it can feel like vegans are at war with non-vegans. However, the more we fight against something, the more we get of that something that we don't want. And it only pushes everyone further down the rabbit hole of what we already believe rather than finding common ground and solutions.

Remember what we discussed in chapter 2 about why people eat animals, dairy and eggs? Keep in mind they are coming from the same place you once did: indoctrination through culture, and fed by misguided information. It's seen as a privilege all over the world to eat like Americans do, and a willful absence of a meat, eggs and dairy-eaters favorite foods is seen on the surface like a self-imposed prison.

What I think we really should attempt to bring about in our day to day lives is constructive conversations about the subject of injustice, because we can all relate to social injustices throughout history. That includes how that injustice makes us feel, as well as a proposed solution. Sometimes, asking the simple question "If you could live healthy and happy without causing violence toward animals, and destruction to our planet, would you?" during conversation can really get people thinking critically about their choices. And sometimes, the conversation stops there. Other times, we want people to desire more information from us on the topic.

I used to work for the number one rock radio station in Hampton Roads, so here is a unique analogy to illustrate how I believe we can get more people to listen to the message of rebellious compassion. Most people are tuned into their favorite radio station, which we will affectionately call WIIFM. Meaning - *What's In It For Me* radio. This is a station we are familiar with because we once listened to it, too. It's the station that gave us everything we wanted to hear and served all of our desires, even when those desires, at times, were superficial. As someone who is already in touch with your Big Why, your commercial for rebellious compassion airs on a different frequency, or station, than your listener is currently on.

You have considered the price that animals and nature pay for your consumer choices, but in order to reach the listeners who haven't yet considered those things, you should first tune into their station (WIIFM radio) and deliver a commercial that keeps them from turning off the radio.

Think of it this way. If you love popular country music and all you listen to is the popular country station, would you expect to ever hear Eminem rap? What would your response be if you did? You'd probably switch the station as soon as possible, shout some expletives at your radio while wondering what the hell just happened.

That is the equivalent of how some well-meaning vegans approach other people in conversation. The non-vegan hasn't been given the chance to decide if they want to hear what the vegan has to say before unsavory things are blurted out.

But, what if while listening to your favorite pop country station, Eminem announced from the studio that he knows this is a bit unorthodox, but he has always been a fan of country. So he and Carrie Underwood did a collaboration and asked that you give it a listen to see what you think. Then, he told you where you can find out more about their album tour if you like what you hear. You might say "no thank you," and switch the station to country classics for a while. Or, most likely, if you like Carrie Underwood, you might stick around to hear the song.

If you stick around to hear it, you may have one of three reactions. You may decide you actually like the sound of it and become a fan. You may decide you hate it and never want to hear it again. Or, you may not love the sound at first...but you keep hearing it everywhere you go so it's beginning to grow on you. If anything, you know the lyrics now because it's become so popular and you hear it everywhere you go.

So, what happens when the well-meaning vegan delivers an unsavory message in conversation from their own frequency without considering their audience? The listener turns the station. They were country, and the vegan broke in with an uninvited Eminem rap.

This can give us some insight into how we can get more people to listen with an open mind. We tune into the listener's current station, which is where we find common ground with the listener, and deliver a nugget of wisdom in a respectful way that won't have them rushing to turn off the radio. They want to know how rejecting their old beliefs can benefit them, and not to be made to feel foolish for their current beliefs about eating animals. So start by being relatable to their current way of thinking. That's where we can build a bridge in our communication with people who are living out their beliefs about eating animals.

Un-Asshole Your Pitch

My heart always sings when I see advocates for rebellious living give voice to the hidden truth about where meat, dairy and eggs come from. However, where I see many well-meaning vegans failing to be heard by the meat eating masses is when they drop the bad news bombs about eating animals, but don't bring that negative energy back up to a positive vibe about how great living a compassionate lifestyle really is for us humans, not just the lower form animals. Some will feverishly shout statements like "meat is murder," thereby coming across pushy and self-righteous. Keep in mind that people don't always remember what you say, but they'll always remember how you made them feel because of what you said. So don't leave them hanging on the bad news. Tell them the good news about why you choose to combat injustice with a plant-exclusive lifestyle.

While not everyone shares an enthusiasm for health, the reality is that many non-vegans share the same fundamental beliefs as vegans do. Most significantly is the belief that we should not inflict suffering and death onto animals unnecessarily. If on any given moment one of us were petting a pig, and then watch someone begin to kick and beat the pig in front of us for no reason, we would try to stop the violence - period. Which is why when we find ourselves at a crossroads between continuing our old habits of contributing to an unjust system, and deciding to take action to eat and live kindly, we want badly to see others make the same *right* choice that we have. We want others to know we are not crazy for taking this path. In fact, we want them to see that the "status quo" are the crazy ones, just like we used to be. And sometimes that need to be *right* works against us in our communication.

We never hear anyone say "The reason I eat meat, cheese and eggs is because I believe that animal suffering and death, and the destruction of our planet's resources, are morally unimportant and harmless events." So why is it then that many non-vegans are quick to defend the status quo, and therefore how do we have more effective conversations about it?

It can be challenging to navigate certain topics around food when our emotions are packaged with the subject matter, and these chance encounters are where we are caught off guard. It can turn out unsavory for both the vegan and the non-vegan inquisitor, just as you've read earlier with Hope and Kris.

That's why I find that using the formula outlined in this chapter for many of the common questions and comments you are likely to hear will help your responses be better received. It involves getting the inquisitor to think critically for themselves. Sometimes, people just don't know how they came to believe what they believe until they are asked. And sometimes, all it takes is for them to hear the words come out of their own mouths about why they believe what they do related to how and why animals are raised for food for the inquisitor to lower their defenses.

Then, you relate to them by saying you used to think or feel the same way, because - hey, you did once upon a time. That piece is critical because we all like people that we can connect with and relate to. Next, you whip 'em up a bad news, good news sandwich, followed by an invitation to learn more.

As a Rebel, I believe you should never ever be afraid to speak about what you know to be true. And when you do, here's an example of a tasty formula to follow. Practice this so you never have to come off as either too passive or too aggressive in your conversations about eating animals again.

Them: "I don't know how you could ever give up cheese. I couldn't!"
You: "What's your understanding of where cheese comes from?"

Why should your response lead with a counter question? Because questions hook the mind by becoming an opportunity for the person to think about what they believe rather than feeling like you are pushing your subjective beliefs onto them. By asking an open ended counter question to their own curious inquiry, we are giving our inquisitor an opportunity to think critically about how they came to believe the very thing that they are questioning. Your goal with the question you choose to counter with is for them to give you an answer that you can relate to. It would go something like this:

Them: "Cheese comes from milk which comes from cows who have to be milked anyway, so I don't see the harm in eating cheese."

Perfect. As a rebel for compassion, you likely used to believe the same thing. And when you make that known, they begin to like and trust you because you have found common ground. Once they know that you understand them and can relate to what they currently believe, think or feel, they will be more open to hearing you on the subject more critically and without undermining your choices. So here's where you relate to them before being the bearer of bad news:

> *You:* **I used to think the same way. But then I learned** *that cow's milk is baby cow growth formula that takes a 65lb baby calf and turns him or her into a 1,600+ pound, four stomached herbivore. And just like human milk is designed by nature for humans, cow's milk is for cows by design, which makes sense that the Physicians Committee for Responsible Medicine claims that the enormous amount of saturated fat in cheese is largely responsible for the obesity epidemic and heart disease.* **And it made me feel** *sad to learn that once the baby calf is born, he or she is taken away from their mom so they can't even nurse from their own mother, and they both cry in anguish for each other for days. The boys become veal, and the girls continue the dairy cycle. Then, the farmer re-impregnates the mom to start the cycle all over again for profit until she is slaughtered for cheap meat.*

Deliver an overview, but try your best not to overdo it as you could lose them before getting to the happy part. You don't want to leave them hanging on just the bad news. You want to show them the hope that being a rebel for compassion provides. They need to understand that there are greener pastures for opting out of such destructive consequences while going through the "inconvenience" of changing their habits completely. They need to see that change is possible for them, so you'll want to address their initial fear about being in lack of foods they love. Always remember to follow the bad news with the good news, and then offer an invitation for them to learn more. In which case you can continue the conversation right then and there if you have permission to, or another time as you both see appropriate. Or you can offer to send a link with additional information that is geared to their primary interest, whether it's health or ethics.

You: "**The good news is** *that there are plenty of delicious plant-based cheeses available in stores so I never feel like I'm missing out on anything. And people love my mac-n-trees recipe made with cheese sauce from cashews. You'd never know it wasn't dairy! I feel much happier and healthier for making the switch to an exclusively plant-based lifestyle. Can I tell you more about this?*"

Often times, the person will follow up with another question, and you can determine more easily if their interest is more in the health or ethical side of things. Once you discover whether it's health, animals, or environment, you can tailor your facts and happy endings accordingly.

But keep in mind that if your why is for the animals, and they are more concerned about their recent heart attack and diabetes, or perhaps the dangerous operational hazards of factory farm workers, then telling them more about animal cruelty until you're blue in the face won't get you very far in this encounter.

Other times, they will indicate that they are not open to further information. Again, pick your battles. You should focus your energy on those who are open to the information. Pushing someone who isn't willing to hear the truth will only make you both frustrated. Fighting only raises people's defenses and encourages them to further reinforce and support what they already believe, and that is not productive for a movement that promotes kindness.

"My only regret is not going vegan sooner. My biggest obstacle to get past was how incredibly hard it would be. About 11 or 12 years ago I got in my mind that it was wrong to kill and eat animals, especially mammals. So I quit eating cows and pigs. But I thought there was no way I could be healthy without eating animal protein, so I only ate birds, fish, and cheese. What a great guy, NOT. In the back of my mind I was feeling guilty as hell by still eating animals. But did it anyway because it would be impossible to not. I wouldn't live a normal life. Wouldn't be able to go out, which is something I did almost every day. I would be skinny and weak. There would be nothing good to eat. Yadayadaya. About 1 year ago my girlfriend and I watched Cowspiracy and we looked at each other and said there is no reason we should still be eating meat, so let's go vegan. We were both like 'oh boy here we go.' We are both the type of person that when we decide to do something we do it. So we were a little worried about going vegan because we both thought it would be so hard and we knew we wouldn't go back to meat after going vegan. So we both go vegan, and it was super easy. There were so many options and our food tastes better than it ever had in our life. We felt healthier than we ever had in our life. Then we took it the next step and went 95% raw, so now we live life 95% raw fruits and vegetables - we feel absolutely great our bodies feel great. We are very healthy and extremely happy. We both feel so good about our decision that we are not harming any animals, we are helping the environment, and all the other many benefits to being vegan.

For once in my life I feel like my life has a real purpose. I dedicate myself to helping animals. And there is some talk of a potential vegan business in the future."

Trevor Dreilich - Venice, FL

Consider Your Audience

Family

Have you ever had the pleasure of trying to convince your family to believe something that is newly important to you when they've known you since you were stuffing toys down your Pampers? And they gave you the 'ol "that's nice, dear." Well, it's likely that this isn't much different.

Now that you have hopped on the wagon to your plant-based paradise and want all your family to jump on the wagon to Veganville with you, you will most likely be met with their concern for your health and wellbeing. Or, some family members might not show a genuine interest in what you have to say, but they are more concerned that you will no longer be eating your favorite casserole that Grandma makes.

So, for family's sake, say as little as necessary in the beginning until they begin to accept that this is not a fad for you. First, inform them of what you will no longer be eating, of course. And be sure to tell them some acceptable alternatives so they won't feel like they don't know how to feed you when you drop by for a meal. Second, consider posting pictures on your social media that they can follow that shows what delicious plant-strong foods you are eating as well as pictures of you being active and healthy. Finally, assure them that while you are still new at it, you are learning more all the time from the doctors who promote a healthy plant-based lifestyle as a way of preventing and reversing chronic disease.

To keep peace in the family, let them come to you with the questions in their own time. And when they do, send them to the experts. Recommend a documentary, book, YouTube video or podcast episode that you believe will answer their immediate concerns. Refer to some that are listed in the Resources section in the back of this book.

If you can't bring yourself to let your sweet grandma see the brutal truth about animals raised for slaughter, watch a more hopeful film with her that focuses on the positive effects of obtaining a meat-free world, like The End of Meat. This will help her to better understand and support your decision and vision for a better world. However, don't expect her to veganize your favorite casserole. Our elders are happily married to their way of doing things, so don't feel disappointed if they don't come around to sharing your vision. Instead, feel happy about the vast changes throughout history that you will get to witness by the time you are their age and the wisdom you will impart on your grandkids someday.

Friends

Let's hope that the company you keep is gentle, understanding and supportive of your newfound love for fruits, vegetables and Beyond Burgers. They may poke fun at you for electing to do a 180 on your diet and your new way of thinking. And, they just might be polite and ask for your blessing to continue eating animals in front of you. Hang in there, and don't blow a gasket on them if your feelings get hurt due to the sensitive subject matter. Just like family, say as little as necessary in the beginning. When they want to know more, send them to the experts by way of video or book, just like with your family.

Since they are your friends, they may be more open to hearing about how you feel on the subject of animal agribusiness. But don't expect them to come to the same conclusions as you. You will likely find yourself in a friendly debate, so invite them to a private viewing of a documentary that shines hope on the issue, like The End of Meat. And be sure to offer a delicious spread of vegan treats as you watch it together, like bbq jackfruit sliders, buffalo cauliflower wings, and hot taco dip.

Hopefully, your friends will remain respectful when you ask them to be. But on the off chance that they aren't, and you feel bad when you are with them, maybe you should reconsider whether or not that is a healthy relationship for you to continue.

New Connections

It's easy for us to assume that because people subconsciously protect themselves with willful ignorance about the plight of animal agriculture that everyone is a dipshit except for you (remember, you were once that dipshit too). This is not the time and place to let your ego take over while shouting "meat is murder." In my experience and taking into account by background in professional communication, that's not the effective way to invite people to listen to your point of view. In fact, it's a surefire way to repulse an otherwise kind-hearted individual whose indoctrination can't let them see the hypocrisy of their actions. If you really want to see more people around you embrace a more compassionate lifestyle, remember to approach every chance encounter with care, concern and curiosity.

Never assume that people's responses to your abstinence from eating animal products is in light of the same information that you have found. Most people have not been exposed to enough of the information that you found compelling enough to make you want to change your habits and thought patterns.

Use every opportunity to keep your negative emotions in check while delivering a small nugget of truth whenever appropriate. So even if you never get the chance to finish your conversation about it, you can rest assure that you have planted a seed in their mind or heart. And you can send up your good vibes into the Universe that you have planted a seed that you hope will take root and grow by the future exposures they will have to healthy and compassionate living out in the world.

Here are three basic principles to follow to help you to keep your negative emotions in check:

Rule #1 - Don't take anything personal. If someone says something hurtful, remember that what people say and do is a projection of their own reality. So learn to be immune to those projections and focus only on your Big Why.

Rule #2 - Speak the truth from your own experience. Refrain from expressing criticisms, judgments, or finding fault with someone. Shine the light on what becoming a rebel for compassion has done for *you*, and not selling them on what it will do for *them*.

Rule #3 - Simply do your best. Your best will change from moment to moment. We go through seasons of change in our knowledge and daily changes in our mood. Do the best you can in the moment you find yourself in. You do not need to be the poster child for veganism or carry the weight of the world on your shoulders. Live your truth and let your actions do the talking.

Keep in mind that no matter who you are communicating with, you are asking them to adopt your idea of a healthier way of life through a more compassionate way of eating. That means you are in a sense asking them to abandon a belief that they currently hold as truth, so be empathetic towards them in your approach. Through asking questions as illustrated above, you can determine how they might be wired to resist your message. Then, that gives you an opportunity to respond in a way that resonates with them as you inform them of what is and what could be.

10

Help New Rebels

"The difference between what we do and what we are capable of doing would suffice to solve most of the world's problems."
Mahatma Gandhi

Whether you help someone in your circle of influence who is open and willing - a parent, grandparent, child, brother, sister, or friend - or you build your own vegan business, helping others unlock their potential to improve their health as well as saving animals is truly the most rewarding aspect of eating like you give a damn. You are already positively influencing other people's decisions through your own actions everywhere you go. Could helping people create transformation be your calling?

One of the best feelings I ever experienced was helping my own mom overcome some debilitating health challenges through a plant-exclusive diet. My mom's story is one that pulls on the heartstrings of everyone who hears it. She has triumphed through physical, mental and emotional challenges that most could never dream of being faced with throughout her life, and most recently one of those challenges was a direct threat to her life: cancer.

Due to prior complications from hernia and cesarean surgeries of the past, and misguided diet and exercise habits over the years, she had been seeing doctors for neuropathy in her legs, bursitis in her knees and hips, fibromyalgia in her shoulders, arthritis in her joints, pains in her abdomen, hypertension, liver disease, and a whole host of other ailments. My mom was only 55 years young and had just entered remission when she found herself needing a walker to get around. And then, tragedy struck. The love of her life who was caring for her better than anyone ever could slipped on ice in the driveway, and became quadriplegic. Then after a hopeful yet difficult year and a half later, he passed away. The emotional and physical pain was too much to bear.

She was no longer capable of taking care of her beautiful property in Tennessee, and had no other choice but to sell her dream home to come live with me and Dave for a while in Florida. And she brought with her all 15 of the medications she was prescribed and took like clockwork, just like the doctor ordered.

My mom understood that Dave and I maintain a compassionate home, meaning that we welcome all things not derived from animals and ensure guests in our home get nothing but kick-ass vegan food during their stay with us.

As a self-proclaimed carnivore and cheese-a-holic, she had become open to seeing how great plant-based food could be while living with us. I took the same intuitive cooking techniques I had learned from her over the years and applied it to a plant-strong menu - most of which contained flavors and textures she was already familiar with. Everything from veganized tacos and stir fry, to "neat loaf" and mac-n-cheese.

Then, when she was ready, we took it to the next level by putting the emphasis on her health for a period of 3 months on a whole foods vegan diet. That meant no mock meats or cheeses, and no processed sugar or white flour so we could restore her gut health.

We introduced juicing to jump start her system, and ate simple plant-strong meals full of colorful fruits, veggies, beans, grains, nuts and seeds as close to whole as mother nature intended. She was amazed at her results. She had lost 50 pounds and experienced a noticeable increase in her energy, stamina, and mental focus (what she called her "fibro fog" had lifted). She stopped suffering from the regular head-aches she used to suffer from, and she realized the swelling in her legs had gone down. And I cried joyfully the first time I saw her leave the house to walk the neighborhood without her walker. She was officially a badass mom who was once again in control of her health and well-being.

After visiting the doctor for blood work, the results were astonishing to both my mom and the doctor. Her liver disease had nearly reversed. And, the doc decided to take her off of two blood pressure medications. A couple months down the road, the doc had removed her from eight more medications.

As she experienced the power of overcoming chronic ill-ness through replacing meat, dairy, and eggs with high nutrient density food, she also picked up on my ethical influences for living vegan as well. She had a clearer conscience and felt happier for learning how to prepare more plant-based meals, as well as finding new alternatives to old animal-centric food traditions.

Perhaps there is someone dear to you that you could help. Just think of the possibility of what could be with what you now know today. Hold that vision, and act on it.

Awaken Your Inner Superhero

A lot of people live life, but pursuing a life of purpose is what truly makes life worth living. Purpose is what drives us to achieve something bigger than we are. For some, their purpose lies in their responsibilities to their family. And for others, purpose is connected to their vocation or meaningful work. Both give life meaning, and if we are sharing our gift of knowledge in the process, we give power to the social cause for compassionate change.

Seeing my mom regain her strength with a lessening of pain, inspiring others to make changes that impact their health and reduce the bloodshed of animals, and creating meaningful work as a vegan health coach showed me just how powerful each of us can be when we put what we've learned to good use.

As a rebel for compassion who is navigating our non-vegan world and inspiring change along the way, you are a pioneer for the largest global social movement in human history. Thousands of people are coming into this new era every day with confusion, habits, health challenges, and questions that you have the ability to help them with. It's time to let your inner rebel to take the reins.

I encourage you to ask this question of yourself: "of all the possible ways to make a difference in the world, how can I make the greatest difference?" In addition to my individual efforts of being a rebel at home, in the workplace and within my circle of influence, after asking that question I felt my purpose rise to the surface. And that purpose involved looking into the many avenues in which I could utilize my knowledge and skills, such as writing this book to help you during your journey.

With the explosion of growth that the plant-based vegan movement is experiencing comes the inevitable learning curve. As you are living and learning as a rebel for compassion, utilize what you've learned by implementing the strategies in this book to be cool and confident about imparting your vegan knowledge to those with an open mind and heart to hear it. They'll come to you when they're ready, so it's not favorable for you to be pushy. Live by example, and when their defenses come down and they're drowning in questions, you'll be there to help.

While rebels are activists by advocating for ethics and personal responsibility to health, you may consider getting involved with organized activism in your local community to expand that message further. Even if organized activism (or organized religion, politics, or sales meetings for that matter) isn't your thing, it can be motivating and uplifting to be in the presence of others vying for the same social change that you want to see in the world. By simply being present at a peaceful demonstration, you are supporting the global movement for peace and compassion that starts at the plate. That ignites and fuels a fire within that translates in your everyday life and interactions, which others around you will pick up on and learn from.

Your new superpower, should you choose to accept it, is that you hold the gift for helping more people along the continuum of making conscious and compassionate choices. Just like respected rebels of our history who were catalysts for change, rebels for compassion don't just ruffle feathers, they make shit happen. Some people like to talk about the problems they see, but rebels take action to solve them.

Seeing as how ditching meat, dairy, and eggs helps to relieve a lot of global problems, and adopting a plant-exclusive lifestyle is pretty easy in most corners of the world while solving many health problems, rebels step up to the spotlight and make this known. And, they make it easy and accessible for anyone who catches the vision and wants to join the mission by helping them along that path.

"I stand as a testimonial to fixing gut issues with a vegan diet. Since I completed the final steps of my transition about 3 months ago by finally giving up my addiction to cheese snacks and cow's milk in my coffee & tea, I have never felt better. I'm off of almost all of my dietary supplements and my 4 Fibercon per day with no ill effects whatsoever. I've weaned myself off of my morning probiotic and I'm able to digest beans with very few issues, and I almost never resort to popping a 'Beano.' All my gut needed was "all plants all the time." So simple, yet I suffered for more than 30 years...SMH! My arthritis, migraines, allergies and general inflammation improved dramatically, too. Stephanie is a fabulous coach and so supportive. If you need help getting to the finish line in your transition to a vegan diet, lean on her! You'll thank yourself for it!"

Rondi Frisch - Vancouver, British Columbia

Bring Your Superpower to the Marketplace

Many people who become committed to the plant-exclusive lifestyle for health and ethical reasons want to express that passion in the form of helping others in a more professional and educational manner. Plant-based enthusiasts become coaches, consultants, culinary chefs, and cruelty-free product curators who start their own practice or sell their own products. For example, Vegan Nutrition Coaches earn their living by guiding their clients on how to transition to and thrive with a healthy plant-based diet.

Now that you're a Rebel for Compassion, and as you get more seasoned and noticed for your noble efforts, you will find that some of the people you meet will want to pick your brain for tips. They'll ask you out for coffee, or to meet for lunch, and after giving your valuable time to them for such a good cause, at the end of the day you've got to provide for you and your family. It's probably a good idea to begin training others, and yourself, to put value on your time and expertise.

Many successful companies who turn a profit and grow operate with a vision of making the world a better place through the products and services they provide. And when you receive validation that you have something valuable to offer people, there's no shame in exchanging that expertise for money, which secures your basic needs and further growing into a bigger and more profitable business that can influence even more positive change in the world.

Individuals everywhere today are feeling the angst of getting a higher education only to end up under a mountain of debt with no promising path to a fulfilling career. Moreover, there are people who have achieved the high status they've worked so hard for, yet they boldly leave their career in pursuit of a purposeful entrepreneurial dream that gives them more freedom and flexibility with their travel and families.

After experiencing the power of being a vegan health coach by helping people meet their health and wellness goals, as well as the freedom and flexibility that comes from being my own boss, my mission today is to create more of that in the world. I provide passionate health enthusiasts with the necessary training they need to confidently build a flexible and profitable business as a Vegan Nutrition Coach. Coaching techniques, balanced nutrition, designing custom menus, developing action plans, and getting clients to the transformation they want are just some of the topics I teach in my Vegan Nutrition Coach Certification course. All of this to better prepare vegan health enthusiasts and aspiring consultants to provide useful service to others interested in the plant-based lifestyle while also earning a healthy profit.

If you're already a health practitioner, heath coach, fitness trainer, or operate any other service based business, or you are passionate about living a vegan lifestyle and aspire to start a business in the plant-based niche with the skills you are proficient in, consider the reach you could have for helping more people adopt a healthy vegan lifestyle by using the power of online influence. The opportunities are 'virtually' endless for you to share your valuable knowledge and skills to a wide audience, and you can monetize them in many ways:

- Start a blog or podcast to document your journey and skills to inspire others and partner with advertisers, or direct your audience to your business offer

- Write and self-publish a book or e-book to document and share your expertise while leveraging it to gain more visibility in your business and compassionate mission

- Host online workshops and webinars to reach a bigger audience and enroll interested people into a 1-on-1 Skype or Zoom session to discuss moving forward with getting them results based on their goals

- Develop a digital course that instructs people step-by-step on how to get the results you have gotten

- Start a YouTube channel and share some general tips from your expertise to gain more visibility and drive more traffic to your website

- Include some affiliate links on your website of products and services your audience would appreciate and is in alignment with your brand while earning a commission

- Start a paid membership site where people can learn from and share openly about the subject of vegan living from their unique perspectives without fear of judgement

- Start an online store on Etsy or EBay to sell your hand-crafted products, and partner with other vegan entrepreneurs online for exposure and to drive traffic to your store

- Develop your signature talk to deliver from stages, and tell the audience how you can help them with your compassionate business or product offer

These are just some low cost and low barrier to entry examples of how you can begin leveraging what you know to help others while simultaneously helping yourself to the freedom and prosperity you deserve while building your legacy and being "the change you wish to see in the world."

If you feel your intuition calling you to this purpose of starting a vegan business, providing plant-based education, or other form of professional advocacy, then start moving toward it today. Write your mission and vision statements, start attending workshops and conferences, network with the people who are already fulfilling their mission, and hire a business coach to help you launch and grow. People need you now more than ever to step into your greatness and sow more seeds of compassion while being a badass leader.

And when you make the decision to move forward with your entrepreneurial advocacy, I want to hear about it. Shoot me a brief message telling me the waves that you will be or are currently making in the world: stephanie@eatinglikeyougiveadamn.com. I love to feature inspiring stories from new influential leaders of compassion like yours on my social media channels!

"The world is a dangerous place, not because of those who do evil, but because of those who look on and do nothing." -Albert Einstein

As you now know, the first steps in creating waves of change is by rejecting the old traditions of consuming animals, combating injustice by revealing a better way to eat and live through your actions, and being the rebel for compassion that is committed to the liberation of all the individuals affected by animal agribusiness: animals and people. When rebels make waves together by thriving in our **health**, our **work**, our **communication**, and our **spirit** for the greater good, the opposition will use it's might to try and regain control of the marketplace. And then, my friends, a revolution will be born. And *we win*.

Resources

I believe the following books, websites, podcasts and blogs will greatly enhance your continued learning about eating like you give a damn in regards to health, environment, animals and our overall connectedness as inhabitants of our shared planet. Many of these are my personal favorites and what I continue to derive inspiration and knowledge from.

Also, join my mailing list at **www.eatinglikeyougiveadamn.com** to keep apprised of further resources which are currently under development to further advance your learning and mission as a Rebel for Compassion.

Plant-Exclusive Nutrition Experts (Books and Websites)

Becoming Vegan: The Complete Reference to Plant-Based Nutrition by Brenda Davis, RD

    www.brendadavisrd.com Brenda Davis is a Registered Dietitian and Nutritionist providing a variety of resources to assist you in making choices that promote and sustain health and well-being, including recipes, articles, FAQ's and videos.

The Cheese Trap: How Breaking a Surprising Addiction Will Help You Lose Weight, Gain Energy and Get Healthy by Neal Barnard, MD

www.pcrm.org Dr. Barnard is the President of The Physicians Committee for Responsible Medicine, which combines the expertise of over 12,000 physicians creating a healthier world through an emphasis on plant-based nutrition and scientific research conducted ethically.

The China Study: The Most Comprehensive Study of Nutrition Ever Conducted and the Startling Implications for Diet, Weight Loss, and Long-Term Health by T. Colin Campbell, MD and Thomas M. Campbell II, MD

www.nutritionstudies.org is where to find out more about Dr. Campbell's work with informational topics on disease, nutrition science, weight loss, and more.

The Complete Idiot's Guide to Plant-Based Nutrition by Julieanna Hever, MS, RD, CPT

www.plantbaseddietitian.com Also known as The Plant-Based Dietitian, Julieanna is a passionate advocate of the miracles associated with following a whole food plant-based diet and the established effects of which provide positive healthful benefits.

Goodbye Lupus: How a Medical Doctor Healed Herself Naturally with Supermarket Foods by Brooke Goldner, MD

www.veganmedicaldoctor.com Dr. Goldner is an internationally-recognized expert in helping patients heal from a variety of chronic disease with plant-based nutrition, and she offers in-home consultations via Skype, Facetime or phone.

How Not To Die: Discover the Foods Scientifically Proven to Prevent and Reverse Disease by Michael Greger, MD

www.nutritionfacts.org is a non-profit organization where Dr. Greger includes a free video library of short, easy to understand explanations of the latest scientific research involving our favorite foods.

Super Immunity: The Essential Nutrition Guide for Boosting Your Body's Defenses to Live Longer, Stronger and Disease Free by Joel Fuhrman, MD

www.drfuhrman.com Best-selling author of Eat to Live and board-certified family physician, Dr. Fuhrman coined the term "Nutritarian" to describe a nutrient-dense eating style, designed to prevent cancer, slow aging, and extend lifespan.

Cookbooks

Betty Goes Vegan: 500 Classic Recipes for the Modern Family by Dan and Annie Shannon

But I Could Never Go Vegan!: 125 Recipes. Zero Excuses. by Kristy Turner

Chocolate-Covered Katie: Over 80 Delicious Recipes That Are Secretly Good for You by Katie Higgins

Eat Vegan on $4 A Day: A Game Plan for the Budget Conscious Cook by Ellen Jaffe Jones

Forks Over Knives - The Cookbook: Over 300 Recipes for Plant-Based Eating All Through the Year by Del Sroufe

The Happy Herbivore Cookbook: Over 175 Delicious Fat-Free and Low-Fat Vegan Recipes by Lindsay Nixon

The Joy of Vegan Baking: The Compassionate Cooks' Traditional Treats and Sinful Sweets by Colleen Patrick-Goudreau

Minimalist Baker's Everyday Cooking: 101 Entirely Plant-based, Mostly Gluten-Free, Easy and Delicious Recipes by Dana Shultz

The No Meat Athlete Cookbook: Whole Food, Plant-Based Recipes to Fuel Your Workouts—and the Rest of Your Life by Matt Frazier and Stepfanie Romine

The Oh She Glows Cookbook: Over 100 Vegan Recipes to Glow from the Inside Out by Angela Liddon

PETA'S Vegan College Cookbook: 275 Easy, Cheap, and Delicious Recipes to Keep You Vegan at School by PETA, With Marta Holmberg and Starza Kolman

Plant-Based on a Budget: Delicious Vegan Recipes for Under $30 a Week, for Less Than 30 Minutes a Meal by Toni Okamoto

Thug Kitchen: Eat Like You Give a F*ck by Michelle Davis and Matt Halloway

Vegan Comfort Classics: 101 Recipes to Feed Your Face by Lauren Toyota

Vegan on the Cheap: Great Recipes and Simple Strategies That Save You Time and Money by Robin Robertson

The Vegan Table: 200 Unforgettable Recipes for Entertaining Every Guest at Every Occasion by Colleen Patrick-Goudreau

Films

Cowspiracy - this Leonardo DiCaprio produced documentary explains how our meat-heavy diets impact everything from climate change and species extinction to land and water wastage. Available on Netflix and at www.cowspiracy.com

Earthlings - this 2005 award-winning documentary narrated by famed actor Joaquin Phoenix explores our relationship with nonhuman animals, including those used in food production. Available in multiple languages. Watch for free at www.nationearth.com

The End of Meat - in this 2018 award-winning documentary, filmmaker Marc Pierschel embarks on a journey to discover what effect a post-meat world would have on the environment, the animals and ourselves. Today, meat producers have launched their own vegan products, 100% vegan supermarkets have opened, and almost every food manufacturer is adding and labeling vegan options. Is this the beginning of the end of meat? Available on Amazon Prime Video, Vimeo and iTunes. View the trailer at www.theendofmeat.com

Fat, Sick and Nearly Dead - this documentary follows Joe Cross, an overweight man suffering from a debilitating autoimmune disease. On a mission to regain his health with juicing and a plant-based diet, he inspires countless others. Available on Netflix, Hulu and at www.fatsickandnearlydead.com

Food, Inc - this 2008 documentary unveiled our nation's food industry, showcasing the unsustainable and inhumane industrial production of meat and the inefficient use of land to grow feed crops for factory-farmed animals. Available on Netflix and Hulu. Learn more at www.takepart.com/foodinc

Forks Over Knives - this film details the health benefits of a plant-based diet, including reduced risk and even reversal of most chronic diseases, including heart disease and cancer. Available on Netflix. Learn more at www.forksoverknives.com/the-film

The Game Changers - this highly anticipated film release of 2019 is executive produced by James Cameron, and tells the story of UFC fighter James Wilks as he travels the world on a quest for the truth behind the world's most dangerous myth: that meat is necessary. Featuring elite athletes, special ops soldiers, visionary scientists, cultural icons, and everyday heroes. Learn more at www.gamechangersmovie.com

Okja - a highly-rated fictional tale of a young girl named Mija and her fight to save her best friend, a "superpig" named Okja, from a powerful corporation that wants to turn her into food. Directed by Bong Joon-Ho and available on Netflix. Learn more at www.facebook.com/OKJAnetflix

Peaceable Kingdom - this award-winning film documents the stories of several people from farming backgrounds who realized that their way of life was not in line with their values of kindness and compassion. Available in multiple languages. Watch for free at www.peaceablekingdomfilm.org

Vegan Everyday Stories - this full-length documentary includes touching interviews with animal rescuers, activists, musicians, doctors, athletes, and more. It traces the personal journeys of four vegans from very different backgrounds. Available for free on YouTube and at www.veganmovie.org

Vegucated - this documentary explores the trials and triumphs of converting to a vegan diet. It follows three meat-and-cheese-loving New Yorkers who agree to adopt a vegan diet for six weeks, and showcases the rapid and at times comedic evolution of these people as they discover that they can change the world one bite at a time. Available on Netflix. Learn more at www.getvegucated.com

What the Health - this film is the groundbreaking follow-up film from the creators of the award-winning documentary Cowspiracy. The film exposes the collusion and corruption in government and big business that is costing us trillions of healthcare dollars, and keeping us sick. Available on Netflix and at www.whatthehealthfilm.com

Modern Animal Agriculture (Websites and Books)

Freefromharm.org - from this website, the Videos tab contains compiled footage from over 150 farm and slaughterhouse investigations, film trailers and scenes, documentaries, and educational presentations about animal agriculture and advocacy.

Humanemyth.org - this website encourages truth, transparency and integrity in animal advocacy while deconstructing the myth of humane animal agriculture.

Meat.org - introduced by Paul McCartney and is said to be the website that the meat industry doesn't want you to see.

Meet Your Meat - this moving narration is accessible on YouTube. It exposes the hidden truth behind factory farming and how meat gets to the table. Narrated by Alec Baldwin.

Slaughterhouse: The Shocking Story of Greed, Neglect, and Inhumane Treatment Inside the US Meat Industry by Gail A. Eisnitz is an investigative report that explores industry facts, and is the first time ever that workers have spoken publicly about what's really taking place behind the closed doors of America's slaughterhouses. The result of these stories gives voice to the animals real life experiences from birth to death.

Why We Love Dogs, Eat Pigs and Wear Cows: An Introduction to Carnism by Melanie Joy, PhD was voted one of the top ten books of 2010 by VegNews Magazine and offers an absorbing look at why and how humans can so wholeheartedly devote ourselves to certain animals and then allow others to suffer needlessly.

Carnism.org is Dr. Joy's website and includes a 17-minute animated video called The Secret Reason We Eat Meat, providing little-known facts about the psychology of eating meat.

Podcasts

Eat for the Planet - Nil Zacharias, author and co-founder of OneGreenPlanet.org, aims to answer the question "how can we eat in a way that nourishes us without starving the planet?" This show features interviews with experts who are redefining the future of food. www.eftp.co/podcast

Food for Thought - voted Favorite Podcast by VegNews magazine readers several years in a row, host and award-winning author Colleen Patrick-Goudreau discusses all aspects of living healthfully and compassionately. www.colleenpatrickgoudreau.com/food-for-thought-podcast

Food Heals - being hailed as "Sex and the City for Food," hosts Allison Melody and Suzy Hardy bring together experts in nutrition, health and healing to teach the best kept secrets to being a hotter, healthier and happier. www.foodhealsnation.com

Main Street Vegan - airing live on Unity Online Radio on Wednesdays at 2pm Central, bestselling author and holistic health counselor Victoria Moran hosts a lively hour devoted to your health, well-being, and living lightly on planet Earth. www.mainstreetvegan.net/category/podcast

No-Bullsh!t Vegan - hosted by Karina Inkster, author and award winning online diet and fitness training creator, whose mandate is to further the vegan cause using scientific truths, not made-up facts. www.karinainkster.com/podcast

No Meat Athlete - hosted by endurance athlete and author Matt Frazier, this podcast provides tools, training tips, recipes, and advice on how to transition to a plant-based diet without the "preaching." www.nomeatathlete.com/radio-archive

Our Hen House - Jasmin Singer and Mariann Sullivan host this unique and fun podcast that focuses on changing the world for animals with interviews including some of the most insightful and inspiring activists and changemakers around. www.ourhenhouse.org/podcast

The Plant Based News Podcast - presented by Robbie Lockie, co-founder of PBN - a content platform and creative agency in London, is aimed at raising consciousness with regards to the environment, health, and animals through insightful interviews. www.plantbasednews.org/tags/podcast

Food Blogs and Vlogs

www.chocolatecoveredkatie.com - this full-time food blogger has provided a top source for healthy sweets and comfort food recipes for people who enjoy delicious desserts and want healthier versions of their favorite foods.

www.theedgyveg.com - Candice Hutchings and James Aita deliver carnivore-approved vegan recipes via their popular

YouTube show, recipe library and food hacks. Decadent desserts, trendy dishes, and fast food favorites – nothing is off-limits.

www.frommybowl.com - Caitlin Shoemaker is passionate about sharing the power of plants with easy-to-follow, healthy, and budget-friendly vegan recipes that are mostly free of gluten, oil, and refined sugar.

www.highcarbhannah.co - High Carb Hannah struggled with depression, weight, drug and alcohol addiction. After finding Dr. McDougall's book *The Starch Solution,* she ended all of her yo-yo weight struggles and now helps others do the same through her food blog and YouTube channel.

www.hotforfoodblog.com - Hot for Food blogger and vlogger, Lauren Toyota, has a knack for creating vegan versions of popular comfort foods like mac and cheese, burgers, caesar salad, and even cheesecake, proving that plant-based diets are far from boring.

www.minimalistbaker.com - Dana is the Minimalist Baker, sharing plant-based recipes that require only 10 ingredients or less, 1 bowl, or 30 minutes or less to prepare. Decadent desserts, hearty entrées and helpful vegan how-to's are just a few of this food bloggers offerings.

www.simnettnutrition.com - Derek Simnett is a Certified Nutritional Practitioner whose YouTube videos are both instructional and inspirational with healthy, wholesome plant-based food and a natural approach to fitness.

www.sweetpotatosoul.com - blogger and vlogger, Jenné Claiborne, was raised in Atlanta, GA and is a trained chef who experienced the healing power of a vegan lifestyle.

Discover cooking videos, healthy eating tips and hundreds of delicious and easy-to-make vegan recipes here.

www.veganyackattack.com - this food blog containing hundreds of plant-based recipes, run by Jackie Sobon, covers everything from indulgent desserts, to healthy dinners, and even raw recipes.

Farm Animal Sanctuary Search and Directory Websites:

Global Federation of Animal Sanctuaries
www.sanctuaryfederation.org/find-a-sanctuary

Your Daily Vegan
www.yourdailyvegan.com/sanctuary-spotlight/sanctuaries

Vegan.com: Making Vegan Easy
www.vegan.com/sanctuaries